Cancer
With
God

CANCER WITH GOD

My
Experience with
Stage 4 Cancer

TERRI LaGUARDIA SCRUGGS

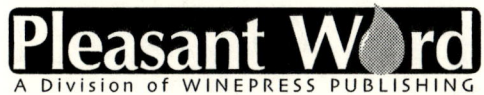
Pleasant Word
A Division of WINEPRESS PUBLISHING

Pleasant Word (a division of WinePress Publishing, PO Box 428, Enumclaw, WA 98022) functions only as book publisher. As such, the ultimate design, content, editorial accuracy, and views expressed or implied in this work are those of the author.

All Scriptures are taken from the Holy Bible, King James Version.

ISBN 1-4141-0472-3
Library of Congress Catalog Card Number: 2005903701

Dedication

This book is lovingly dedicated to my big sister, Christine LaGuardia Phillips, who died of breast cancer in 1975 at the age of twenty-two. I miss you!

Table of Contents

Introduction

In 1975, when I was eighteen years old, my sister died from breast cancer. She was twenty-two. The doctors told me I was likely to get cancer, too, since I was the younger sibling closest to her in age. Sure enough, in early April of 2003, I was diagnosed with squamous cell vulvar cancer. It had already spread to the lymph nodes and was in stage IV.

I fought this cancer with chemotherapy, radiation, and the grace of God. There were blood transfusions, infections, physical therapy, surgery, and a miracle.

If there is anything in the world I hate, it's cancer. In my mind, cancer is evil. It can break your body and your emotions. It can kill your spirit. It can even destroy your soul . . . if you don't fight it.

My intention in writing this is to be an inspiration for those who have cancer now or have had it in the past. I hope this book will help you deal with the effects of this terrible disease. I can show you how to handle it with a positive outlook, even while keeping the realities in mind.

Chapter 1

Cancer Tears:
They told me I have cancer!

One day, when I was busy building my goals,
I looked to my side and saw them crashing down.
I looked up and said, "God, please don't let this be true."
Yet when I looked around, I learned my life had changed.

In April of 2003, doctors told me I had squamous cell vulvar cancer. They said they were sure I would live; they just didn't know how much of my body would survive.

I love my heavenly Father, and I knew He would take care of me. Yet I had to acknowledge there was that chance I would not win this battle.

Now, a positive attitude has been part of my personality my whole life, and I didn't want anyone to know how devastated I was. In private, however, I cried tears that could have made rivers, and I prayed to my dear Lord for mercy.

I told my family and friends I was fine. They knew I wasn't.

Unreal Death

My life has taken a twist and I am afraid.
I set many goals, but I was not prepared.
They said I have cancer, the disease of death.
I fear for my body; it seems to have no worth.

Must I face destruction? How should I prepare?
My insides are shaking and my mind is in fear.
My sister died of cancer; is that my fate too?
This has to be a bad dream. It just cannot be true.

I do not want to believe that this cancer is inside me.
But the tumor is real, and the depth of the pain is mighty.
I find resolution in facing the fact that I am dying.
It is like an earthquake, and I have nowhere to run.

*Have not I commanded thee? Be strong and of a good cour-
age; be not afraid, neither be thou dismayed: for the Lord
thy God is with thee whithersoever thou goest.*
—Joshua 1:9

What could possibly have led up to all this? There'd been
warnings, but I didn't want to see them. I had never heard
of vulvar cancer. I thought I had a simple yeast infection.

I am an entrepreneur, so I really did not have time to
sit in a doctor's office. I figured I could take care of this
problem with an over-the-counter remedy. So I tried one,
but the infected area began to swell and bleed. That's when
I started to wonder if it might be some kind of cancer.

I went online to see if cancer was possible in this area. After many days of searching, I came across a blurb about vulvar cancer. I began to worry.

I hadn't been to the doctor for anything in a couple of years and had moved to a new state since then. I hadn't even taken the time to find a new doctor. But now, I needed to talk to someone.

My New Journey

I fought the fear for months.
I could not recognize the reality,
Thinking it must be something else.
It cannot be happening.

Then one day I bled so much
that the truth gripped my body.
I shed tears for hours
Before I considered sharing this tragedy.

I reached for my husband's hand,
finally accommodating the cancer.
My new journey began as I told him
All that I had kept under cover.

I saw fear in his eyes as he asked me
Why I had quietly lingered.
I told him it was only a couple of months ago
When it started.

The relief in feeling his concern
Helped me feel at peace.
I finally had someone to lean on
Through the uncertainties.

I heard him crying during the night,
And it touched my heart.
This man cared so dearly,
He was afraid for us to part.

*Now the God of hope fill you with all joy and peace in be-
lieving, that ye may abound in hope, through the power of
the Holy Ghost.*
—Romans 15:13

My parents pulled some strings and got me in to see their family doctor the next day. She was not sure what my problem was, so she referred me to a gynecologist. He wouldn't tell me what he thought, but he referred me to a cancer doctor.

Neither of these first two doctors had done a biopsy. So I figured the referral to a cancer doctor was simply a precaution.

Four weeks after I'd gone to the family doctor, I saw the cancer doctor. After looking at the affected area, she told me it looked like cancer. She ordered a biopsy.

The results confirmed her theory. She set me up for radiation and chemotherapy treatments right away. I went home that day with a fear in my heart that I had never known before.

Only My Tears

I hide in my corner, not talking to anybody,
Sitting in tears, my body soaked with misery.
I tremble in fear, thinking there is no hope.
Shaking extends all over me, trying to escape.

Where do I turn? How do I ask for assistance?
My heart breaks at the thought of this disease.
To share with someone would be so easy,
If only I could open up and talk about this worry.

I need someone who can relate to why I suffer alone,
Someone who can sense what I do, who feels the pain.
I can't escape my doubts; the stress builds up inside.
I spend hours wanting to cry and find a place to hide.

*According to my earnest expectation and my hope, that in
nothing I shall be ashamed, but that with all boldness, as
always, so now also Christ shall be magnified in my body,
whether it be by life, or by death.*
—Philippians 1:20

We set up my doctor appointments and scheduled a CAT
scan for the next day. My fear grew stronger as I realized
that this cancer may have spread to my lymph nodes and
could be all over my body.

When I received the results, I learned that the cancer
was in my lymph nodes, but only in the immediate area.
My chances looked somewhat better.

The following week I saw my radiologist and he set up
a plan of attack. I was to have treatments five days a week

for a total of twenty-nine treatments, starting the following Monday.

That Wednesday I went to see my chemotherapy doctor. He performed the only blood test anyone had given me to that point. Then he set up an additional plan of attack. I was to have a twenty-minute drip of cisplatin and a ninety-six-hour drip of 5-FU during the first and last weeks of radiation therapy. He told me that within three weeks all of the hair on my head would be gone.

Soon after getting home, the nurse from my chemo doctor's office called and told me I had to check into the hospital immediately, as my red blood cell count was low. I asked how low, and she told me 6.2. I went to the hospital and received two units of blood.

That night, at home, I thought over everything the doctors had told me. The truth began to sink in. If the therapy didn't work, there was a good chance that my rectum, bladder, uterus, cervix, lower colon, clitoris, and vagina would need to be removed. One doctor had told me I might not survive.

Everything I'd experienced during the past week engulfed my mind. I broke down.

Why Me?

I quietly held close the recollections of my existence.
The trauma hit me. Why do I have this horrifying disease?
I am not a mean person; I did not do anything wrong.
Why would this happen when my love for God is strong?

16

I do not deserve this. Listen to me! Take notice!
I want to live longer, not die like this.
I do not want to walk this path ahead of me.
I refuse to accept the growth inside my body.

If I recognize it, then it will become a reality,
An ugly truth determined to rupture my very being.
I do not want to know it; it does not really exist.
Go away! Just go away! Leave my presence now!

*Call unto me, and I will answer thee, and show thee great
and mighty things, which thou knowest not.*
—Jeremiah 33:3

The cancer did not go away.

I went in for radiation the following week. Before I could start the chemotherapy, I had to have another two-unit blood transfusion and have a Portacath installed.

I quickly lost all the dignity I had ever known. This was not due to the people who performed the therapy. They were perfect to me. My dignity was lost because of the particular area where the tumor was. Each visit involved exposing it, and there was no way around that.

Every day I prayed to God, asking Him to remove this cancer from my body. I didn't think He was listening.

Cancer had not only changed my routine, it also changed my outlook on life.

I started taking all kinds of medicines; mainly, dicloxacillin, diphenoxy, silver sulfa cream for radiation burn, Kytril, hydrocodone, Promethazine, Percocet, Coumadin, daily vitamins, vitamin C, bromelains, cephalexin, and ferrous sulfate.

What Is Normal?

It took over my life; each day I felt a new horror.
The anguish was inside me, changing my existence forever.
I no longer knew what normal meant, or how I was to be.
My life is a horror story built upon an agonizing reality.

The doctors and nurses became my new friends.
Their offices were my daily hangout; yet I was not lost.
Daily I talked to my heavenly Father, who held my hand.
I felt safe as He crumbled my painful mountain.

I needed to cross a stormy ocean to escape the agony.
My Lord lifted me up into the sea of tranquility.
Normal became a lesson in trusting during adversity.
I held His hand tightly and gave Him all that hurt me.

*He shall cover thee with his feathers, and under his wings
shalt thou trust: his truth shall be thy shield and buckler.*
—Psalm 91:4

A Godly Story

Some sections of the stadium are full of weeds. Other sections are ragged and do not resemble their past. The last section has the look of a new creation.

This stadium reminded me of life. We forge through it with determination, breaking all the rules in the name of our goals. We look back at all we have accomplished on our own and see a meadow of fascinating-looking plants, growing everywhere with no visible end. Some are climbing, others crawling and stumbling over one another with no apparent motivation.

We wonder what happened to all those goals, why none of them was a complete success. Then we look around and realize that our life really has no meaning. Just like the crumbled part of the stadium, our lives do not resemble the future that our birth ordained.

It is hard to cross the road we cannot see. Yet some of us do it. We turn our backs on the disappointments and look up for the truth.

It takes some time to learn how to keep our hands in His and not question His direction. But eventually we learn to love it, and our souls leap for joy. We greet the last section of our lives with a new spirit. He not only gives us a new start, but He wipes out all the weeds and destruction. We are newborns in His eyes, and our lives have only just begun!

And Joshua said unto the people, Sanctify yourselves: for to morrow the Lord will do wonders among you.
                                                    —Joshua 3:5

Chapter 2

A Day With Cancer:
One day of the struggle

I dropped my life to fight this battle of terror.
No smiles to ease my pain, no road for the escape.
I cried for hours, not knowing what the future held.
I prayed for another chance to turn my life around.

As I woke up to a new day, the pain and seriousness of cancer filled my mind. My eyes opened to a world of emptiness. I had lost every physical aspect my life had ever known.

I looked up to the ceiling in my bedroom and closed my eyes to spend some time with my God. My husband slept beside me, so I spoke to my Lord in silence.

My words to Him were full of honesty. "Dear Father, please help me. Take the cancer away."

I recognized that without Him this disease would have encased my mind in sorrow. I told Him how important He was to me.

21

"Thank You for being with me throughout the past few weeks. I have needed You to keep the cancer from discouraging me. You have helped me to live with the reality that I am a victim of cancer."

The shock of this statement suddenly overwhelmed me.

"I have cancer. Oh, my dear God, I have cancer! Please just take it from me. It hurts so badly."

Tears soaked my face as I felt a deep, disparaging agony embrace my body. I reached to my bedside table and grabbed two pain pills. I took them with a sip of water. The cancer hurt so much!

I knew the day needed to go on, so I slowly climbed out of bed. It hurt just to move. *Will this ever end?*

Throughout the previous weeks I had learned to be a casualty of cancer. The pain of getting out of bed was only the beginning of my new routine. Even the many trips I took to the bathroom involved sheer agony from the effects of the radiation treatments on my skin. My clothes made for more pain, and walking became a task. At times, the tumor felt like a collection of knives cutting through my body.

Knives

The knives dig deep into me,
Piercing my interior identity,
Taking twists that turn and twirl.
It reaches in depths immeasurable.

My soul is screaming out,
"Make it stop, just make it stop!"

22

I could not get away from the pain.
It did not matter how far I ran.

Please do not stab me again!
Oh, why is this happening?
The realm of my body throbs.
It suffers countless jabs.

But his flesh upon him shall have pain, and his soul within him shall mourn.

—Job 14:22

I needed to get ready for my radiation therapy. I would be going in for chemotherapy after the radiation therapy was over. They were on opposite sides of the hospital, so we had to drive from one to the other.

My skin was full of blisters and I had uncontrollable bouts with diarrhea. Just getting dressed hurt, never mind the pain of walking and riding in the car. My life was pure torment, but I was determined to get through another day.

My Therapy

It burnt through my skin, flew through my inner being,
Breaking apart the invader, cleansing it from my body.
The radiation hurts my skin, frying my casing to a peel,
Making my organs revolt; yet without it is fate's seal.

If I were lying in fire, it could not hurt worse.
Yet never could a bandage have such results!
When today's radiation was complete, it was time
To go to the other side and get my chemotherapy done.

Chemicals flowing through me, trying to fight the cancer,
Taking no prisoners and blindly clearing the corridor.
The other chairs are full with other victims of the disease,
A room of bald heads and faces blemished with sadness.

*Why is my pain perpetual, and my wound incurable, which
refuseth to be healed? wilt thou be altogether unto me as a
liar, and as waters that fail?*
                                                    —Jeremiah 15:18

After a day filled with therapy, I came home, looking
forward to resting in my own chair. The home nurse had to
connect me to my ninety-six-hour chemo bag. I hate carry-
ing that thing around. I was always afraid it would tangle
and rip away from my port.

It felt good to be home and have no more medical people
around me. The day had been quite painful. I decided to
take a few pain pills and go into my peaceful little world.

Escape

This cannot be real; I must be in a hospital, sleeping.
I am deep in unconsciousness, not truly with the living.
That's it! I'm not here! This is just a make-believe life.
I do not really have cancer; it's all just a false strife.

The pain feels genuine, but I do not believe it is so.
I am just lying in bed, letting my imagination go.
The house is a spaceship; I use it to flee the pain.
I fly through the universe, avoiding all the rain.

I fly through God's painless place in the heavens.
It's peaceful – there's no sound, no hurt in my dreams.
I fly within the stars and see endless hope and glee.
I escape from the pain and find a new reality.

And I saw a new heaven and a new earth: for the first heaven and the first earth were passed away; and there was no more sea.

—Revelation 21:1

I awoke from my nap a few hours before bedtime. It had been a tiring day. My body hurt and the therapy had made me weak.

I've had it with this cancer. I just want to run away.

If there'd been any way to escape this, I would have taken it.

Today's Storm

Today is not a good day. My mind is exhausted; I feel sad.
There are reasons to feel this way, and it is getting so bad!
I need someone to talk to, but no one will understand.
These feelings are like a bottle exploding in my hand.

I need a release, a source that will not judge my emotions,
I need time to express what is deep in my mind's vision.

I gather my things to run for cover, looking for a hero.
The skies blacken and drain; the winds begin to blow.

Can I hold on alone? No. I need someone to take my hand,
Taking me from danger - to the light at the tunnel's end.
A hand holds mine and someone speaks my name.
He is pulling me out of the storm to safety again.

*Stand in awe, and sin not: commune with your own heart
upon your bed, and be still.*
—Psalm 4:4

I put on my nightgown, took my medicine, and climbed
into bed. It was time to talk to my Father.

"Hi God! Thank You for giving me another day to spend
on this earth. Thank You for enabling the therapy to shrink
my tumor. I love You so much! I don't know what I would
do without You."

My God is an awesome God and I love spending my last
minutes awake talking to Him.

"It's been a hard day, Father, and I'm exhausted. This
cancer is agonizing! Please take it away from me."

There were days when I wanted to give up on the cancer. The therapy caused more hurt than the cancer did. If
it weren't for my heavenly Father, I could never have made
it through.

"Thank You, Father, for giving me the strength I need
to conquer my daily walk with this cancer."

Clouds

I must cross the water; the waves are crashing in my face.
The sky is dark and busy; the wind encompasses my eyes.
I am standing in a doorway and cannot see past the storm.

Every step brings me sorrow; the pain breaks my progress.
Each step is agony; the clouds fill me with darkness.
Yet I must go forward because my life is beyond the sea.

*Cause me to hear thy lovingkindness in the morning; for in
thee do I trust: cause me to know the way wherein I should
walk; for I lift up my soul unto thee.*
—Psalm 143:8

Christine, one of my older sisters, died of breast cancer
in 1975, the year I graduated from high school. She died on
our mother's birthday. She and I are two of nine children
in our family. My parents are Tom and Kathryn; and my
siblings are Mike, Kathy, Larry, Christine, Shirley, Tommy,
Mary Ann and Virginia. I love all of my family members
very much.

After Christine died, a cancer center was built in our
hometown to help others who suffer with the disease. The
Christine LaGuardia Phillips Cancer Center is a compre-
hensive provider of oncology care. It is the leading cancer
center in the state in the new treatment for prostate cancer. It provides diagnosis, treatment, and support, using
state-of-the-art equipment and techniques.

27

This is where I received all my therapy. Christine would have liked knowing that her name was contributing to the welfare of cancer victims.

I remember my mother telling me a story about when Christine was a teenager and had just learned about cancer in a class at school. It upset her very much, and she told our mother about it, saying that someday she was going to go into research to help find a cure for it. Now, because of her cancer, there is an awesome cancer center, in her birthplace, that helps people from all over the country every day.

Christine was four years older than I was, and the closest big sister I had to my age. Losing her was a major blow to our entire family. She was the only sister I had with whom I shared my entire life. Even through her cancer, she was always there for me, as I tried to be for her. She will always be in my heart.

When I was about three years old, she would come into the bedroom I shared with my little sister and pray with us. She taught me how important prayer is and how loving Jesus is. Christine nurtured my Christian life. The way I miss her is unexplainable with mere words. But I can say, without a doubt, that she touched my life in a way no one else ever has.

Christine

My sister, I miss you!
I need you with me, to give me your shoulder for rest.
Cancer took you away so young - your future lost.
You are in heaven, getting ready for us to come in,
I look forward to the day when I run to hug you again.

Christine, I love you!
I want to phone you and have a sisterly chat.
I need to share my life with you as we did in the past.
Let's talk over lunch; I want your guidance again.
You are the only person who could ease my mind.

My sister, I remember you!
I kneel and pray daily, as you taught me to do.
I pleaded for God to remove the cancerous tumor.
God sent me a special gift as I finished my prayer.
I asked Him to let you pray for His healing power.

Christine, I miss your smile!
After my prayer, I felt a gentle touch and looked around.
I saw you kneeling by my side, with a smile on your face.
With a glow from heaven, you looked in my eyes and left.
I received a peace that assured me I would win the fight.

I will never forget the night God blessed me with a choir of angels led by my sister.

For he shall give his angels charge over thee, to keep thee in all thy ways.
—Psalm 91:11

A Godly Story

Once upon a time, there was a little girl named Teeny. She had lots of sisters and brothers who kept her life full of activity. She was having a wonderful time living her life.

Then one day doctors came and stood beside her sandbox. They had awful news that changed her life forever.

Teeny ran home to her mother and father for comfort. They held her closely and encouraged her to fight it. So she did. While the doctors put her through agonizing therapy, she talked to God about living longer. When the doctors told her tomorrow would never come, God comforted her soul.

The therapy was hard on her, yet she fought with all her heart. Her parents suffered every step of the way with her, trying to find some way to keep her with them.

Still, the day came when God assembled the angels and opened His gates for her arrival. Her family assembled around her as she shared her love for them.

Suddenly a glow filled her eyes and a smile brightened her face. The pain had gone.

She left her family behind for her eternal mansion in heaven. There she found her sandbox and began living again.

Teeny always takes time to pray for the family and friends who have not yet come home.

Chapter 3

Failure:
The therapy did not get it all

The fight was hard and brought me down to earth.
I shed my dignity and lost my pride in the struggle.
Then I looked up past the rubble and saw the tunnel's end.
Yet I had not won the battle; my life would never be the same.

That awful summer, the radiation therapy took away
every part of my dignity. My strength was gone and my will
to live had lessened. Those last days of therapy took every
bit of my life away from me.

But I was thankful that I was still alive.

Skin

My skin is on fire. It is peeling from my body.
It hurts so badly and I cannot stand the throbbing.
Every blister accumulates on top of another.
One will disappear to emerge into several more.

The heat from the area encases my entire being.
The pain is taking over; I cannot stop the agony.
They told me radiation would be helpful.
How can this misery have a label of gentle?

As I realize that I am dying from the exterior,
It peels and then scabs and I go back for more.
The swelling, the fire, the excruciating pain;
I find myself exhausted and deeply sentient.

*My flesh is clothed with worms and clods of dust; my skin
is broken, and become loathsome.*
                                                                    —Job 7:5

As hard as I tried, I could not hold in the grief anymore. The pain was more than I could handle. Embarrassment encompassed each day, whether I was receiving therapy or just trying to deal with each moment.

On some days I had to wait a few minutes to see the doctor. Those minutes seemed like hours. I would be crying hard by the time he came in.

Throughout the last week of therapy, I cried uncontrollably every day. I usually hold in my tears, since I don't like people to see me crying. This cancer changed that.

My intestines were in disarray from the radiation, and diarrhea sent me to the bathroom constantly. I had to wear adult diapers because I couldn't completely control myself. My entire body felt like it was on fire.

I didn't like myself anymore.

Breaking My Spirit

I cannot take it anymore. Make it leave me alone!
My body is falling apart; I just cannot function.
I want to give up and quit participating in sanguinity.
It hurts to move around; I do not want to be living.

It keeps growing in me, crossing my spirit with anguish,
Not caring about the future, making me feel worthless.
The chemicals in me are trying to eradicate the cancer,
Yet I am afraid that they are destroying my total character.

My heart wants to continue, but my body is in tears.
I know the therapy is defeating the evil intruder,
Yet I don't know how I can continue with this choice.
It has destroyed the good along with the heinous.

I was not in safety, neither had I rest, neither was I quiet;
yet trouble came.
—Job 3:26

I finally got to the end of the therapy. That summer some
good things had happened, including the fact that none of
my hair fell out. More important, the tumor shrank! But I
still needed the operation.

My cancer doctor checked out all the information concerning my therapy and looked at my tumor. The big smile
on her face was quite a relief to me! She told me she should
definitely be able to get it all with surgery.

Yes!

However, there was a catch. They had to take out more than just the tumor. The removal of my left vulva, along with my clitoris, was also necessary. There was some question as to whether all or part of my vagina and bladder would need to be removed. And I would have to undergo extensive plastic surgery.

My heart sank. I asked if there was any way we could do some additional radiation therapy to get more of it. She explained that the therapy had shrunk the tumor very well and totally removed the cancer in the lymph nodes in my right groin area. But it was still in the lymph nodes in my left groin.

I was going to live. Yet what kind of life was I facing? There would be no more radiation therapy in my future. I decided to accept my new life. At least I had hope!

My Resolve

There are times when I feel all alone.
It hurts, down deep in my bones.
I have a resolve burning my spirit.
I must turn my head to the hurt.

Do not tell me it will be all right.
Maybe it will, maybe it will not.
I know that the potential is there;
Nonetheless, only my soul is aware.

My heart aches with deep throbs.
The pain deep within me is absorbed.
I must not let it give me apprehension.
I cannot let it grasp my inner being.

Failure: The therapy did not get it all

O remember that my life is wind: mine eye shall no more see good.

—Job 7:7

A Godly Story

Once upon a time, there was a little girl who loved walking in the park. She went there every chance she had and walked for hours on end. Her parents always looked for her there when she was late.

It was such fun walking around the park! There were trees as tall as the sky and flowers blooming so proudly that their smell filled the air when she walked past them. Sometimes she skipped through the majesty of nature.

Friends invited her to play with them, and she ran to them and enjoyed the companionship they shared.

One day she fell while running and broke her leg. A doctor put a cast on it and told her it would take a few months to heal. She kept going back to the park to walk, but it wasn't the same on crutches and in a wheelchair.

The little girl became very sad and cried a lot. She still went to the park, where she watched her friends playing, and imagined herself having fun with them.

When the day came for the cast to come off, the little girl was so excited! Her friends were waiting in the park for her to come play with them.

The doctor took off the cast and told her to sit still while he talked to her mother. They came back with sad looks on their faces. Her leg was better, but it hadn't healed completely. She was going to need surgery, and the doctor wasn't sure the little girl would ever walk again.

35

The little girl began to cry, not knowing if she would ever be able to skip through the park again.

(This story is continued in Chapter 5.)

Cast thy burden upon the Lord, and he shall sustain thee: he shall never suffer the righteous to be moved.

—Psalm 55:22

Chapter 4

Truth:

My body was about to be torn apart

I took a deep breath, and tears soaked my face.
My body did not want to accept what the future held.
My soul insisted on faith, to believe the truth.
I believed, but never believed enough to let go.

After I got home from finding out what needed to taken from me, I went to a room and cried alone.

A week later, I visited the plastic surgeon. He told me the repairs would be extensive. He said they would remove a piece of my stomach to use for the missing skin and that grafts would come from my right leg. I would need to come back to redo the initial surgery at least three times, since it would be difficult for the new skin to stay in place in that area. Each stay in the hospital would last at least three weeks.

I listened to everything he said and signed all the paperwork. My husband brought me home and I read every information sheet the doctor had given me.

I cried as I considered my future. I was going to live, but my life was never going to be the same. I looked up to my heavenly Father and began praying.

"Father, I'm scared. I need Your help. This is going to be so hard! I don't want to face this; it's awful! This is not the kind of life I want.

"Lord, you know I have always loved You. Now I need strength and determination and tranquility, which I can only get from You. Please touch my soul and give me Your hand.

"There are times in the past when I've fallen. Even in those times, my heart looked up to You. Without You I am nothing. Touch me, Lord. This is going to be so hard! I'm glad I have You."

I beseech thee, O Lord, remember now how I have walked before thee in truth and with a perfect heart, and have done that which is good in thy sight.
—2 Kings 20:3

God had mightily blessed me, because the therapy did more than the doctors thought it would. But I could not face what was about to be done to me. I needed to let the doctors rip my body up, discarding parts that had always been useful to me. How was I supposed to live without all of me? How would I function? I had to spend the next six months in bed, and then how would I deal with the rest of my life?

I wanted to wake up and be a five-year-old, securely in my parents' home, and not have to deal with this reality. I began praying.

"Oh, God, this is not what I want my future to be like. You are holy; You are the Almighty. And Lord, I do appreciate what You've done for me, how You helped the therapy to work against all odds.

"I know it's only in You that I can find the hope I need to go on. Please touch me with Your grace, for I need this blessing. I feel lost and I cannot understand why this has happened to me. Yet I know, dear Lord, that this is not as bad as it could be.

"Jesus, I know Your suffering was far worse than what I have to bear. Thank You for giving me Your blood so I can live the life I have. Lord, You are faithful and Your mercy endures forever. I need You now more than ever. Hold me!"

For the hope which is laid up for you in heaven, whereof ye heard before in the word of the truth of the gospel.
—Colossians 1:5

As I was praying, I suddenly realized that God had always been right by my side. Every single step of my life, He had put up with my goodness and my wrongdoings. He helped me get up every time I fell. He had placed me in a family and around friends who cared for me. So what was there to worry about? Through Him, I knew I could make something good come out of all this. I should be thanking Him for all He'd done for me.

I reached into my soul and went back to my heavenly Father in prayer.

"I'm sorry, Lord, for all the griping I've done this year. My heart knows that it's all about You. You are everything, and I need You. Search my soul, look into my heart, and see my love.

"I give You all my praise. Hallelujah! You are my God. Throughout my life, You have given me a great reality. I know I can make it through whatever the future holds, and that no matter what comes my way, You will be by my side.

"You are so awesome, God! My life has always been in Your hands. You have taken such good care of me throughout my life. You are my King, my Father, my Savior, my Lord, and my Strength. Thank You for loving me so much that You gave Your dear Son to save me."

For this cause also thank we God without ceasing, because, when ye received the word of God which ye heard of us, ye received it not as the word of men, but as it is in truth, the word of God, which effectually worketh also in you that believe.
—1 Thessalonians 2:13

My prayers were sincere. Yet I suddenly realized that I'd never given God all of me. I thought about how much He loved me, with such an endless love that I could not ever understand it.

At that moment, He brought such a peace to my heart that I fell to my knees in reverence to Him.

"Oh, heavenly Father, I am so sorry I haven't served You as I should. I've spent my life setting silly goals that meant nothing in Your sight. I've been serving myself instead of

You. How could I do that? I'm sorry. When I get past this surgery and recovery, I promise to serve You better.

"You are so glorious, dear Lord! I want to be the person You want me to be. I have never fully given myself to You, never really served You. I don't understand how I could have neglected You like I have. These last few months have made me realize that life needs to be lived!

"The only way I can live the rest of my life is through You, dear Lord. Oh, Father, I ask that You release Satan from my heart and sanctify me. I give You all my worries and all my pain because I know You care. You can take care of me in a way no one else understands. I love You, Lord. Amen."

Humble yourselves therefore under the mighty hand of God, that he may exalt you in due time: casting all your care upon him; for he careth for you.

—1 Peter 5:6-7

A Godly Story

Once upon a time, a star was in charge of a whole galaxy. Every day it would shine its light over every planet in its galaxy. It was an awesome star, and planets in other galaxies wondered what this light was all about.

One day a large comet flew into this galaxy. It had heard of this remarkable star and wanted to get rid of it. The comet had a flame of its own and did not want anyone to have this star's light.

As it flew by each planet on its way to the star, these planets tried to stop it. Nevertheless, the comet made it safely to the star.

41

"Your light will become darkness," the comet yelled.

The star just looked at the comet and smiled.

The comet, which was almost the size of the star, summoned all of its power and ran right into the star. The star began to tear apart, with pieces of it flying throughout the universe.

The comet had a smirk on its face, thinking it had stopped the light from shining.

Suddenly the comet realized that all the planets in the universe were singing joyous songs. The entire universe began to light up. The star had turned the comet's evil plans into a universe full of grace. Every galaxy now had its own light shining brightly upon its planets.

The comet tried to get away from the light, but the brightness overtook it. Finally, the comet let go of its flame and accepted the light from the star.

The comet and the planets lived happily within the warmth of the star that had spread its light throughout the universe.

The morning stars sang together, and all the sons of God shouted for joy.

—Job 38:7

Chapter 5

My Prayer:
I gave my life to God and accepted His will

My last day of what was left of normal came upon me.
I sat down by myself and gave my entire future away.
I looked up to the Lord my God and asked for a miracle.
I gave my life to Him and accepted His will.

On the day before the surgery I was terrified. My life was about to change again. Everything God had given me that I took for granted was about to be taken. I spent the day in prayer, asking God to help me get through the surgery all right and to help me deal with my new life.

I prepared for the ordeal by shaving my legs, doing my nails, washing clothes, packing my gowns and slippers, cleaning the house, and making sure someone knew where I kept my life insurance papers. Throughout it all, I was in prayer.

"Hi God; please be with me today as I prepare for my surgery. Give me the strength I need to take care of the things

I need to do. Take the worries of tomorrow away from me so I can function today. Do not leave my side. I need You to hold me today, for I am worried.

"See the tears soaking my face, oh, Lord? I need You to cleanse my heart. Everything I know is about to change, and I'm frightened. I cannot believe this is happening tomorrow! I need Your strength. I keep checking the tumor, hoping it has gone, but it's still there.

"Lord, I know there's no turning back. I have to face the fact that my body is in turmoil. In the morning, the doctors will cut and remove parts of me I want to keep. Please help me adjust to the horrible thing that is about to happen."

Be careful for nothing; but in every thing by prayer and supplication with thanksgiving let your requests be made known unto God. And the peace of God, which passeth all understanding, shall keep your hearts and minds through Christ Jesus.

—Philippians 4:6-7

The day passed very quickly, and soon I was preparing for sleep. I pulled my covers down and put on my night-gown. I was alone in my bedroom, so I sat down and pleaded with God to help me.

"Oh, God, the day I have dreaded all year long is almost here. Please God, just hold me. Hold me! I need to feel Your touch. I'm so scared. My future is not the one I want. This is awful! If there was a place to run and hide, I would go there this very instant.

"Oh, Father, there are things in my past of which I am so ashamed. I know You have already forgiven them. But I need to tell You again that I'm sorry for all the sins of my past. If I could do it all over again for You, things would be different.

"As I sit here today, Lord, I want to give You my future, as bad as it is. I want to be more of a child to You, to share Your light in my innocence. Father, I know my life is going to be hard. I give you no blame, only glory for how You gave this much to me."

He asked life of thee, and thou gavest it him, even length of days for ever and ever.
—Psalm 21:4

After a few moments of silence, I began thinking over my life. God had always been there for me, no matter how rebellious I was.

I remembered when I was fourteen years old and He asked me to serve Him. I prayed about it for days and really considered doing it. But there was no opportunity for a woman to be a minister or priest, so I let it go.

When I was twenty-four years old, I almost died while having a C-section. I saw the pathway to the glorious gates of heaven. My grandmother had left for heaven two weeks earlier, and He let her tell me, as I was running toward the Light, "Your girls need you!"

The next thing I remember is waking up and finding out that my third daughter was waiting for me to hold her.

Two years later I had a child who was stillborn. Her name is Kelly. She's in heaven. She had several problems, including hydrocephalus, cleft lip, missing fingers and toes, and more. I believe it was a blessing that God took her home instead of letting her live a miserable life with a deformed mind and body.

Two weeks after Kelly left us, my youngest daughter had breathing problems. She was twenty-two months old and I thought her asthma was acting up. I took her to the emergency room. It turned out that she had a growth in her throat. The doctors were going to have to do emergency surgery, as this sac was full of poisonous fluid and if it burst on its own, it could kill her.

I thought I was about to lose another child.

The doctor ordered X-rays and conducted an examination. Then my little girl went to surgery.

When the doctor came out, he was smiling. He told me a miracle had just happened. When the surgeons went to remove the growth, they found nothing there. They redid the X-rays, and sure enough, the growth was gone!

God has done many other miraculous things for my family, my friends, and me in the past.

I sat in silence for a long time, thinking about my trust in God. I checked for the tumor; it was still there, the same size it was when I last saw my cancer doctor. I looked up to heaven as I had never done before.

"Oh, Father, You have given me so much. Hallelujah! You are incredible, and I cannot express my awe of You. Jesus, look down on me tonight and listen to my cry.

You showed me today that my love for You is missing complete trust. Tonight I am finally aware. You have shown me the light. Right now, this very moment, I am going to give You my total trust. I don't know why I never gave it to You before, but that day is gone. I have always believed in You. Now Satan's hold is gone; my trust is full.

"Father, I ask You, in the name of Your dear Son and my precious Savior, Jesus Christ, please have mercy on my soul and heal my body before the surgery tomorrow. I am frightened of what my future will be without a miracle from You. Please take this tumor from my body so there will be no need for plastic surgery."

The sorrows of death compassed me, and the pains of hell gat hold upon me: I found trouble and sorrow. Then called I upon the name of the Lord; O Lord, I beseech thee, deliver my soul.

—Psalm 116:3-4

My prayers had turned around. I began the day accepting whatever the doctors were going to do to my body and asking God to give me the strength to deal with the aftermath. I ended the day trusting in God's will. I had given my life to Him.

"Father, I plead with You, in the name of Jesus, Your loving Son, to have mercy on me and grant my request for a miracle. I trust You. I know You will do whatever is best for me. This very moment I give my life to You to do with as You want. My faith has never been stronger than it is right now, Lord. But I am still scared. Please help me!

"Jesus, please take this request to Your righteous Father. I believe in You, Jesus. You know that. Thank You for coming to earth and dying for my sins. I need Your help tonight. Oh, Jesus, please help me! I am so scared. Please, Jesus, talk to our Father for me. Tell Him that I'm scared and that I need help. I want the tumor to disappear. Please, Jesus, help me tonight!

"Dear Father, I give my life, my future, completely to You. Thank You, Father, and thank You, Jesus, for taking such good care of me.

"I know the decision is Yours, and my desires may not be Your will. I accept whatever decision You have made. I understand that removing this tumor may not be what You want for me. But Father, I ask for this miracle in the name of my dear Savior, Jesus Christ. Thank You, Jesus. Thank You, Father. Amen."

For every one that asketh receiveth; and he that seeketh findeth; and to him that knocketh it shall be opened.
—Matthew 7:8

A Godly Story *(continued from Chapter Three)*

The little girl had broken her leg. The doctors had told her they needed to operate and she may never be able to walk again. Her heart sank within her, as she loved to walk and run in the park with her friends.

The night before the surgery, her big sister came to her bedroom and closed the door. She sat beside her and told her, "I know you believe in Jesus and what He did for us. Now I need you to look to His Father and give Him your complete trust. He can help the operation to work out so that you can walk and run again. Reach deep into your soul. He is there waiting for you. Give Him every fear you have and He will replace them with total love."

The little girl looked up to her big sister and smiled. She then closed her eyes, reached for her sister's hands, and gave God every one of her desires and fears. God took them and gave her His immaculate grace.

A few months later the little girl was at the park, smelling the richness of the flowers she was running past. She looked up to her heavenly Father and said, "It's all about You, Lord!"

Cause me to hear thy lovingkindness in the morning; for in thee do I trust: cause me to know the way wherein I should walk; for I lift up my soul unto thee.

—Psalm 143:8

Chapter 6

Restoration:
I let the doctors take control

I slept that night better than I had all year.
The fight had been long and I tried to calm my fear.
The next morning I took the road to the life of change.
I let my doctor take my body in her hands to repair.

When I went to sleep that night, I found a peaceful rest for the first time all year. God had touched me with a peace that filled my soul and calmed my pain.

Tranquility

After my prayer was over, I climbed into my bed.
I looked up and smiled at my Father, whom I loved.
I closed my eyes and fell asleep, feeling His presence
Taking care of my pain and holding me in His arms.

I felt like a baby cuddled in the arms of her mother.
I had not a care in the world, an innocent spectator.

The pain was gone and the tears stayed within.
I peacefully drifted off into a world that was calm.

I do not remember the dreams I had that night.
They should have been about winning the fight.
God was with me throughout my battle with cancer.
Only He had control over the ultimate encounter.

*I will both lay me down in peace, and sleep: for thou, Lord,
only makest me dwell in safety.*
—Psalm 4:8

Now, as I think over all the struggle and pain that led me to that night in peace with God, I can see how He was right by my side the entire way.

When I woke up the morning of the surgery, I thought of what my day was going to be like. The fears came back for a moment, so I started the day with prayer to my heavenly Father.

"Hi God; please be with me today. I'm scared and I need Your loving hand. Last night I found peace in Your loving arms. Today I need You more than ever.

"I love You so much! I cannot live without You by my side. You are my almighty Lord, my holy Father, and my Savior. You are everything I know and all that encompasses my life. Without You, I would die from loneliness.

"I beg You, Lord, to take away any fears left in me. I know there is no reason to worry with You here. Hold my hand this morning and help me get ready. I'm scared and I need You to keep Your peace within me. Amen."

Behold, I have graven thee upon the palms of my hands; thy walls are continually before me.

—Isaiah 49:16

When it was time to get ready for the surgery, I took the last shower I expected to have for a long time. I quickly dressed and was ready to go to the hospital.

A Life Of Change

It was time to take that step into reality,
Time to depend on the Trust I hold on to.
I will put my life into the hands of strangers.
My body will forget the knowledge of the years.

This road to change is not one I want to travel on.
Yet I must be strong and cross it with determination.
I know that with God by my side things will be easier.
He cares for me in such a way I know I can persevere.

It is hard to look into a future of transformation.
My life will be different than it was before.
My heart desires a connection with my spirit.
I by no means want to part with this moment.

That their hearts might be comforted, being knit together in love, and unto all riches of the full assurance of understanding, to the acknowledgement of the mystery of God, and of the Father, and of Christ; in whom are hid all the treasures of wisdom and knowledge.

—Colossians 2:2-3

My family met me at the hospital. I checked in and a nurse took me to my room. She gave me drugs to calm me and a gown to change into. I changed and got ready for the inevitable.

In a few minutes, the nurse came back in and told me someone would be coming to get me for the operation in five minutes.

I went to the bathroom one last time. While in there, I remembered that I had not checked for the tumor since waking up. I had asked God for a miracle, and I needed to see if He answered that prayer.

I checked for the tumor where I knew it to be, but I couldn't feel it! I checked all around where it always was again, yet I couldn't find it. I then checked my lymph nodes – they were still swollen. I went back to the tumor. I thought that it must have moved. Yet it's been in that same place for months now, why would it move overnight? I looked up to God and asked Him, "Did you take the tumor away?" Tears fell down my face.

I was eager to run out the door to my family and tell them that God took the tumor away. I hesitated, realizing that I needed the doctor to confirm that it was gone before I got everyone excited about it. In my mind, it could have moved further inside of me, where I couldn't feel it. I decided not to tell my family. I would just go to the surgery and tell the doctor before she put me under. She could then check and confirm that the tumor was truly gone!

When I walked out, I saw my family sitting there, looking sad. I joked a bit about how I wouldn't be able to dance a jig for a while. Then I danced in circles for them, laughing all the while.

They all thought I was being silly, but I was actually excited at the thought that God may have removed my tumor!

A nurse came into my room to take me to surgery. As I was being taken to the operating room, I asked if I would be seeing the doctor before surgery. They told me that I would, so I contemplated in my mind how I would say, "I think that the tumor is gone!"

While going through the halls of the hospital, however, I worried about the doctor telling me that the tumor was still there. I didn't want to think about the operation, nor the aftermath. The thought of the doctor cutting into me, and the mess my body was going to be after the surgery – it was more than I could handle. Yet, what if the doctor confirmed that the tumor truly was gone?

I don't remember seeing the doctor before I went into the operating room. I must have been drugged up pretty good, and I went under before I knew what was happening.

The Operation

Traveling towards the surgery was effectively eased
By thoughts reaching out to the new hope I discovered.
We reached the surgery room, and I looked for my doctor.
I needed her to verify that the tumor was not there.

They gave me medicine and told me to take it easy.
I asked about the doctor, and they said she was on her way.
I imagined telling her, "The tumor is gone!" with a smile,
And seeing her joyful face after confirming the miracle.

I smiled and asked my Heavenly Father to be by my side.
He is my Rock, He is faithful, He is forever my Lord.
Without Him, I am nothing; with Him, I am a conqueror!
With His strength, I have found my ultimate cover!

Suddenly I began getting questions from the nurses,
Asking about previous operations and their effects.
I told them about a C-section that I woke up during.
I must have fallen asleep before the end of the questioning.

*Thou hast turned for me my mourning into dancing: thou
hast put off my sackcloth, and girded me with gladness; To
the end that my glory may sing praise to thee, and not be
silent. O LORD my God, I will give thanks unto thee for
ever.*

—Psalm 30:11-12

A Godly Story

Once upon a time, there was a small town, east of the
coast, where everything was purple. The sky was purple,
the seas were purple, the grass was purple, the animals were
purple, even the people were purple. It was quite a sight
to see! But it was hard to distinguish the beauty of shapes
because all the purple mixed everything together.

One day a visitor came to town. His skin was brown,
and he had a yellow car, blue clothes, and a green hat.

Everyone in the town of Purple was shocked! They
began whispering among themselves.

"Where did this person come from?"

"He must be from outer space because he is so different."

The brown man heard this and smiled. He told them he was from a little town a few miles away and that most of the world was the same as he was. He asked if they watched TV. They said no. The screens were all purple and they could not see anything through the purple.

He told them he knew how to make their town normal. The purple people thought they were normal, but as the man described the beauty of colors, they began listening to him.

Then he told them of the truth. He told them that the transformation of the world would happen before their eyes if they would only have faith.

Some of the purple people did not believe him and just walked away. Yet most stayed and were excited about what he was teaching them.

"It's through our total belief in the truth that we are able to release ourselves to His care," the man said. "Our faith can only be nurtured through the power of the Holy Spirit."

He told them that God would give them the ability to see other colors if they would just let Him. Some said there was no way this could happen. But the man pointed out to them that they were seeing his different colors. He said that was because he was sharing his love for God with them.

He urged them to share their love for God with him. "Your faith should not rest on human wisdom," he told them, "but on the power of God."

They asked him to tell them more about God. He told them that God loved each one of them so much that He sacrificed His only Son to save them.

Purple people all around began falling on their knees and praising their heavenly Father. Their love for God spread all over town, and most of the purple turn into a vast array of gorgeous colors.

Others began seeing the love of God all over town, and they accepted Him into their lives too. Soon the town was renamed Rainbow. And they all lived happily ever after.

I was with you in weakness, and in fear, and in much trembling. And my speech and my preaching was not with enticing words of man's wisdom, but in demonstration of the Spirit and of power: that your faith should not stand in the wisdom of men, but in the power of God. Howbeit we speak wisdom among them that are perfect: yet not the wisdom of this world, nor of the princes of this world, that come to nought: but we speak the wisdom of God in a mystery, even the hidden wisdom, which God ordained before the world unto our glory: which none of the princes of this world knew: for had they known it, they would not have crucified the Lord of glory. But as it is written, Eye hath not seen, nor ear heard, neither have entered into the heart of man, the things which God hath prepared for them that love him. But God hath revealed them unto us by his Spirit: for the Spirit searcheth all things, yea, the deep things of God.
—1 Corinthians 2:3-10

Chapter 7

The Miracle:
The beginning of all I know

What I had not known was that God repaired me first.
Yes! That day was the beginning of all I know.
The months to come were a different kind of battle.
I had to climb out of the woods and into the sunshine.

The moment I opened my eyes after surgery, the nurse at my bedside placed her hand on my arm and told me the doctors did not have to do what they had planned. She said they had to remove ten lymph nodes, but the tumor was gone. They had cancelled the plastic surgeon.

I touched my stomach, looking for the stitches, but there weren't any! I looked at her and asked if she was kidding. She said, "No kidding! You are a living miracle."

Could this be true, or had I died and gone to heaven? Or maybe I was just dreaming!

It Is A Miracle

I fell hard and needed help getting up.
I looked to my family and friends for help.
They ran to my rescue and reached for my hand.
My heart felt stronger having them around.

I went to the doctors and did everything they said.
I spent days getting fried, drugged, and poisoned.
After the therapy, my doctor was set to cut into me.
She stopped when she could not find the tumor.

The invasive surgery was no longer required.
They'd called the plastic surgeon and canceled.
The tumor had disappeared; no longer was it in the way.
The doctors were shocked at what happened that day.

If I'd been awake, I would have shouted out with a shrill,
"It's gone! It's gone! God gave me a miracle!"
My soul is full of joy; my heart is cleansed.
My eyes do believe; my life has become humbled.

Bless the Lord, O my soul: and all that is within me, bless
his holy name. Bless the Lord, O my soul, and forget not all
his benefits: who forgiveth all thine iniquities; who healeth
all thy diseases.
—Psalm 103:1-3

The hospital staff took me back to my room, where my family was standing outside. They all looked so sad. Obviously they hadn't heard the news!
"You all don't know, do you?"

My husband came to my side. He told me they'd heard the surgery went well and had gone faster than it was supposed to. I looked across the hall and saw my doctor walking toward my parents. I smiled at my husband and told him to go listen to what she had to tell everyone.

As I was wheeled into my room, the doctor spoke to my family out in the hallway. I heard their shouts of excitement.

Everyone came into my room, and their frowns had turned upside down! My doctor gave me the official word, and I praised my dear heavenly Father. Everyone stayed for a long while as I went in and out of consciousness.

It was a special day of celebration that I will never forget. I was even able to pray with some of my family members.

After they had all left and the nurses were done with their duties regarding me, I looked up to my Lord and thanked Him for at least the fiftieth time that day. I told Him I wanted to always follow His path. I closed my eyes, put out my hand, and said, "Take my hand, Lord, and lead me wherever You think I should go. I am Your servant, and I'll spend the rest of my days serving You the best I can. I love You, Father. I love You so much! Thank You for this miracle. Thank You!"

That day, August 8, 2003, was the first day of my life. I have always believed in miracles, but when a miracle touches someone the way this one did me, it is a humbling experience. That evening I humbled myself before my dear Father more than I have ever done in my life. I went to sleep thanking Him with tears of joy.

New Life

Birds are outside my window.
Their singing appears to flow.
A joy has filled my heart
As they soar and tweet.

God must have sent the flocks
To help open my sleepy eyes,
To let me know that a new day
Has stirred toward my way.

An extraordinary day full of life
That has said good-bye to strife.
Their sweet song overwhelms me,
Making me want to be all I can be.

I know what needs to be completed.
I must share His splendor with the world.
My eyes are opening to His plan.
I have found a purpose to sustain.

*For thou hast delivered my soul from death, mine eyes from
tears, and my feet from falling. I will walk before the Lord
in the land of the living.*
—Psalm 116:8-9

The fight was finally over, and the path God had me on
was becoming clearer to me. I can never forget how cancer
almost destroyed me and what God did for me all along the
way to recovery. He touched me with His glorious grace and
changed my life forever.

The Field

A field crossed in front of my path and it hurt my soul.
I stopped at a flood that ran down the gutter so bold.
The storm rumbled above the horizon, darkening the sky.
I looked at the chaos and could not let this pain go by.

I fell on my knees, face down, - asking for mercy.
Not knowing what, nor where, life was for me.
No one being should be so close to my interior person,
Since it will end with damage over my inner dominion.

I never imagined a path so hard, so full of strife.
I want the right to grasp for the full length of my life.
Then I crossed the rainbow flying over the horizon
My soul is humbled beyond the eyes of my imagination.

*Grace be unto you, and peace, from God our Father, and
from the Lord Jesus Christ.*
                                                —Philippians 1:2

A Godly Story

There once was a lonely girl who looked up to the stars,
amazed at their vast brightness. As she sat in a meadow on
the revolving earth, she began to realize what a great creation
was a part of her existence. She looked at the multi-colored
tulips that glowed in the moonlight. She observed the trees
bowing in the warm breeze that touched her face.

The enormous sky once again caught her attention as
thoughts of the Creator filled her mind. The glory of all He
had placed there for her to enjoy encased her sight. Prayers

filled the air—the joyous sound of praises for His tender canvas of love.

A star suddenly flew across the heavens. In the silence, a heartfelt sigh engulfed the darkness. The little girl looked to the mountaintops and saw the sun's immaculate rays across its peak. A new day was in its infancy.

I love the Lord, because he hath heard my voice and my supplications. Because he hath inclined his ear unto me, therefore will I call upon him as long as I live. The sorrows of death compassed me, and the pains of hell gat hold upon me: I found trouble and sorrow. Then called I upon the name of the Lord; O Lord, I beseech thee, deliver my soul. Gracious is the Lord, and righteous; yea, our God is merciful. The Lord preserveth the simple: I was brought low, and he helped me. Return unto thy rest, O my soul; for the Lord hath dealt bountifully with thee. For thou hast delivered my soul from death, mine eyes from tears, and my feet from falling. I will walk before the Lord in the land of the living. I believed, therefore have I spoken: I was greatly afflicted: I said in my haste, All men are liars. What shall I render unto the Lord for all his benefits toward me? I will take the cup of salvation, and call upon the name of the Lord. I will pay my vows unto the Lord now in the presence of all his people. Precious in the sight of the Lord is the death of his saints. O Lord, truly I am thy servant; I am thy servant, and the son of thine handmaid: thou hast loosed my bonds. I will offer to thee the sacrifice of thanksgiving, and will call upon the name of the Lord. I will pay my vows unto the Lord now in the presence of all his people. In the courts of the Lord's house, in the midst of thee, O Jerusalem. Praise ye the Lord.

—Psalm 116

Chapter 8

My Support:
My family was my lifeline

I look around and see the support He has given me:
Caring, loving people who share my love for Him.
Yet never have I been able to thank Him enough
For this miracle that gave me a new life with Him.

On February 7, 1957, God blessed me with a wonderful family. My parents saw to it that I grew up in a good Christian home with values as strong as stone. The foundation of my faith is sure because of the love for God that my parents taught me.

From this foundation, I have grown closer to God as my life has proceeded. This foothold brought my soul to attention the day God had mercy on me and blessed me with an enormous miracle.

Throughout the trial of cancer I suffered, my family was right by my side. I thank God for surrounding me with such a realm of love. I thank each of my family members for being who they are.

Attachments

I was walking in the moonlit night,
Analyzing the seriousness of my fight.
As I crossed the tulip-lined bridge,
I looked up to a beautiful ridge.
My mind began to drift into a smile.

I remember the innocence of my youth,
How my parents gave me details of the truth.
Teachers taught me the importance of the golden rule.
Playmates showed me the strength in companionship.
I tried to live by these lessons of life.

As I came upon a meadow, I stopped and looked about.
The flowers were full of life and the sky smiling with light.
I sat down in the richness of the green meadow.
I began to look at what I have in my heart now.
My senses soared with the freshness of life.

I praised my heavenly Father for blessing me
By giving my soul a life that will live through eternity,
With parents who have never stopped being my example
And a family who have been by my side through it all.
Friends who have passed by are attached forevermore.

*Trust in the Lord with all thine heart; and lean not unto thine
own understanding. In all thy ways acknowledge him, and
he shall direct thy paths.*
                                        —Proverbs 3:5-6

My Support: My family was my lifeline

My children—Amanda, Katie, Theresa, and Matthew—mean the world to me, more than I could possibly express. I did my best to bring them up to love God. I made many mistakes along the way, but I pray they will face their Creator as I have.

Each of my children has his or her own personality and life. From my girls, who were by my side during the cancer, I saw a depth of concern that gave me a stronger will to live.

My daughter Katie was born by emergency C-section because she was breech. She had stuck her foot out while I was in labor. I knew then that this little girl was going to keep me jumping. And she sure has! She has grown into a strong, willful woman and I am proud of how far she has come.

The following is a note Katie wrote concerning what she was feeling while I was fighting the cancer.

When my mom was diagnosed with cancer, I tried to pretend it wasn't really happening. If I let myself think about it too hard, I felt as if I would not be able to bear it. I tried to support her by calling often and letting her know how much I loved her. It was almost as if I felt guilty in some way for not being able to help her get better physically.

Throughout most of her treatment, I kept my fears at bay and hoped for the best. There were many times when I wondered what would happen if she didn't survive this. I mean, nobody in our bloodline had ever survived cancer before. Why would she be any different?

Losing my mother became an issue I had to face head on, and it wasn't easy. I love my mother very, very, very much, and even today, when I think of losing her, my eyes fill with tears. I cannot begin to think of how painful that day will be.

Her chemo was very hard for her since it was mixed in with her radiation treatment. She never did lose her hair, though, and everyone I have ever told this to has been amazed, especially people who have loved ones in remission. I guess I should have taken this as a good sign, but I could not think on the situation for very long.

The day before her surgery, I called her to let her know that no matter what happened, if she was given the choice to leave this life, under no circumstances was she allowed to go. Selfishly, I told her I needed her, that I could not live without her, and that she could not leave me yet. She promised me she would not go anywhere, and though I was still afraid, somehow that made me feel better. I mean, she'd promised, right? Moreover, if God tried to take her, she would tell Him no because she knew how much I needed her.

The morning of her surgery, I slept so I would not have to feel the anxiety of waiting for the outcome. I arrived at the hospital, with my little sister, just as she was taken into her room from recovery. My family members, who had been waiting at the hospital all morning, gave me these looks like I didn't care about her or something. Little did they know I cared the most, and would have been a wreck in that waiting room all day.

But none of that mattered because the doctor had good news. The surgery had gone better than expected, and somehow her tumor had completely disappeared. She was going to be fine. She'd kept her promise!

—Katie La Guardia

The last enemy that shall be destroyed is death.

—1 Corinthians 15:26

My Support: My family was my lifeline

Amanda is my oldest daughter. I am proud of the woman she has become.

She is the ideal big sister. I watch how she deals with her younger siblings. They know they can always go to her when there's a problem, or just to share sisterly time.

This is what Amanda wrote about my cancer.

When I found out my mother had cancer, I was very upset and concerned about her welfare. The discovery that her cancer had advanced into the fourth stage devastated me. I thought about the stories I had heard of her sister and the futile struggles of my godmother when they faced similar news. I thought my mother would be the next in the family to succumb to this disease and I was not happy about it, to say the least. In fact I was very scared for my mother and worried about how she would deal with all the pain and hardship she would soon have to endure.

During the treatments, I visited her often. We discussed her medications and how she was feeling. Many family members came by and dropped off food and gifts to help my mother and stepfather through this difficult period.

I enjoyed going to visit with my mother every week before the cancer, and I was happy that I could continue that during her treatments.

As the success of her treatments progressed, surgery loamed closer. Initially, they told us that my mother would need a major surgery involving difficult, prolonged, and painful cosmetic adjustments. This was a scary prospect for my mother and the entire family, as it would mean she would be confined to bed for a long period of time and possibly have to undergo further surgeries, not to mention the person-ally devastating side effects. I was very worried about her during this time.

When she went into surgery, I was in the hospital room with my grandparents and other family members throughout the day. She completed the surgery early, and we were all surprised to find out the tumor had completely subsided and that no major surgery was needed. I believe this was due to the great ability of her doctors and the intensive treatment she received, as well as her strong, positive attitude throughout treatment.

When she got cancer, I felt as though I would lose the person I often turned to when I felt the need to vent, or just talk about things that were going on in my life. When my mother came through the cancer, I felt very thankful that she gave such a brave and enduring fight and won. I also felt lucky that I could keep my mother with me for at least a few more decades so we could continue to spend time together and she could get to know her future grandchildren.

The cancer was difficult for my mother, and in the aftermath of facing her own mortality, she is bringing a stronger belief system into her life, which will provide more stability if she ever has to face death again. I believe this is a good thing for her, and I hope her life goes in the direction she has always hoped for herself.

—Amanda La Guardia Healey

Surely goodness and mercy shall follow me all the days of my life: and I will dwell in the house of the Lord for ever.
—Psalm 23:6

My stepson was in Iraq, proudly fighting for our country, while I was suffering through my therapy. I am proud of what he did for America, yet relieved to have him back home.

Following is what he gave me concerning my cancer.

When I first learned of my mother's cancer, I was overseas in the army. I had received permission to make a phone call home, and I figured it would be like any other phone call. When I received the news of the cancer, I was shocked.

My parents' optimism slightly relieved me, but I was still very worried and concerned. I immediately began to pray that everything would be okay. It was humbling to me because I thought being in Iraq was bad, yet my problems suddenly paled in comparison.

I am tremendously grateful and relieved that everything turned out okay. God really does answer prayers!

—Matthew Scruggs

I will praise the Lord according to his righteousness: and will sing praise to the name of the Lord most high.

—Psalm 7:17

Theresa is my youngest daughter. She has a heart of gold and an imagination that could move ships! She has grown into a wonderful woman. She keeps her values and never lets anyone else be in control of her. Her determination to be the best at what she does makes me proud.

This is Theresa's look at my summer with cancer.

It's hard to say when I first realized my mother had cancer. Of course, I knew she did, but when did I realize it? Was it at the beginning, when she was in pain and could barely walk? Maybe it was when she called me to say that the doctor found her test sample to be malignant. Or was it when I saw her come home from her first chemo treatment, tired and weak to the point of collapse? I still do not know. Did she ever have cancer?

I do not like admitting it, and I certainly do not like talking about it, but that is part of how I cope with things.

The summer she was going through all this, our family was shaken to the core. What would we do without her? She was the glue in our family, the reason to wake up every morning. The one person you knew you could always have, the one who would always be there. What would happen if all of a sudden she was gone?

No. She can't have cancer. But she did. The best course of action in my strange little mind was to ignore it and make believe she was just sick, plain and simple.

I was home for the better part of every day that summer, so I saw her ill, drugged up, and in continuous pain. I couldn't deal with it. I had to get out. Therefore, I did the only thing I could do: I left. I went in other rooms; I went to my sister's apartment. I did anything to avoid watching my mother's downfall, because in my mind, it wasn't really happening.

On some days, I tried to keep her company in the den and watch TV, just to be around her. I attempted to carry on like normal and hold regular conversations, but she would always fall asleep or nod off. I felt selfish for being mad at her for such a thing, so I just left the room and didn't come back unless she called me there. She was not the only one in pain, but not many people seemed to realize this.

The worst thing I have ever done in my life was to not donate blood for her. But I wasn't self-centered; I was scared. What if something went wrong, and it was my blood that killed her? I could not live with myself. I knew the risks involved with getting blood from non-family members, but I couldn't bring myself to hurt her with my own. So I just didn't do it.

I know there are many arguments against me in this situation, but I'm the one who knows why I do things. Sure, I regret it, but I had my reasons—twisted as they may have been.

This was my mother, not someone I barely knew. And she was dying. Sometimes I felt like I should resent her for having cancer since I would probably have it one day too. And I don't want it. God, I really don't want it. Yet because of genetics, it will most likely happen. It's like a time bomb, ticking. Every strange thing I find on my body now scares me to death, even when it is the most harmless thing possible.

I don't want to be unhealthy because of things I cannot help. I don't want to be different. I don't want to be stared at and pitied.

So I was not about to pity my mother for having it. I wanted to give her the same courtesy I want when it one day happens to me. Therefore, I treated her as if nothing was different. I pretended she just left the house every morning for meetings and slept all day because she was tired.

I wondered when her hair would start falling out from the chemo treatment. I even told her, when she needed to start wearing a wig, not to take it off when I was around. I didn't want to see her without hair, because that would have made it all too real.

Luckily, by some huge stroke of fate, her hair never did fall out—which was amazing. I had hoped it wouldn't. I guess you really do get some things you pray for.

One day, I went with my mother to the doctor's office for somewhat of a final analysis of what would have to be done in surgery. I don't know whether she was overly confident about her pending results or what, but she let me come back with her and my stepfather to hear the news first hand.

That's when it hit me. No fewer than four organs were to be removed. And there was a good chance she'd have to live with tubes hanging out of her for the rest of her life.

She tried and tried to see if there was anything else that could be done: more chemo, more radiation. She was willing to go through all that pain all over again just so she could live a normal life, with everything intact. The final answer was no, and she was forced to deal with it. She was devastated.

On the way down to the car, we were in the elevator alone and I felt I should say something. I was never good at talking to people like that. It's just not part of how I work, I guess. But I needed to say something to make her feel better. So I made a feeble attempt at consoling her. I said, "The doctor said a lot of people can live fine without some of it."

Then my mom said, "But I can't."

I didn't know what else to say.

The surgery came and went. I arrived at the hospital with one of my sisters and found my mother had been taken into her room. She was barely able to talk, but we waited anyway. There were a lot of family members there.

When I heard from the surgeon that there was no cancer left in her when they went in, for some reason I wasn't even surprised. Everyone kept going on and on about a miracle, but to me, it was just what was supposed to happen to begin with. I was never optimistic, and I didn't give myself the chance to be pessimistic, but somewhere in my heart of hearts, I knew she was going to be okay. Everything happens for a reason.

Sometimes you just have to die a little to live a little better.

—Theresa La Guardia

Bless the Lord, O my soul. O Lord my God, thou art very great; thou art clothed with honour and majesty. Who coverest thyself with light as with a garment: who stretchest out the heavens like a curtain: who layeth the beams of his chambers in the waters: who maketh the clouds his chariot: who walketh upon the wings of the wind.

—Psalm 104:1-3

My children amaze me with the individual ways they show love. This poem is for them, because death really was not an option.

Death Was Not An Option

I had cancer - yet my main fear was not of the disease.
I did not tell the entire prognosis to those closest to me.
My children have always depended on their mother;
They knew I would always be there, that my love was true.

This place required explanation that crossed the line.
I had to convince my family that I would be fine.
I told them about it on the phone, to lessen the blow.
I asked God to cover them with His feathers of gold.

Knowing the fear in my heart would arouse their worry,
I told those I loved that this cancer fight would be easy.
I decided not to let my children know that I might depart.
It kept an alternative alive that would calm their hearts.

I will praise thee, O Lord my God, with all my heart: and I will glorify thy name for evermore. For great is thy mercy toward me: and thou hast delivered my soul from the lowest hell.

—Psalm 86:12-13

My husband, Warren, was the constant that kept me moving through the whole arena of therapy. He was always right there for me, taking care of everything I required. He exemplifies what the words *man* and *husband* mean. He gave me all the support and love I needed while I had cancer. He has always been that way, and I know he loves me.

Every morning, he took me to the radiation treatments, sitting with me and helping me whenever I needed him. He cleaned up all my messes, learned to take care of the house, and made sure my needs were met.

Below are his words about what he went through while I had cancer.

I remember the moment Terri told me something wasn't right. I was scared, but to tell the truth, I was also a little angry that she let it go for so long. The night she told me she thought she may have cancer, I wanted to believe otherwise, and I told her so. But I had an uneasy feeling she might be right.

It was one of the longest nights I have experienced in my forty-seven years.

I got over the anger part pretty quickly and we started doing what we could to find out what was going on.

This began many trips to doctors. It was hard to watch her decline as time went on. We went from arriving at the offices talking and kidding around to, toward the end of her therapy, just focusing on getting to the doctor's office as quickly as possible, as she was in total agony just riding in the car. It was a tough time for us all.

While Terri was going through this, our son went off to war in Iraq with the Army's fourth infantry.

One of the things that bothered me the most was that I felt so helpless. Sometimes the feeling of helplessness was more than I could bear. I wanted to take the cancer away from Terri, to be with our son while he was in danger, and to convince our girls that as bad as everything was, it was all going to be okay. Just your typical husband/father stuff, right?

But nothing was routine anymore. I was scared of losing her. I knew the cancer was bad. It hurt so much to watch her be in such pain, and I was glad for her when the medication knocked her out. I figured she wasn't hurting while she was asleep, and I wanted so much for her to stop hurting.

I did what I could to make her comfortable and tried to keep her spirits up. That is somewhat odd, because Terri is the most positive-minded person I have ever known. She will never let anything stand in her way of doing something she wants to do. I believe that is one of the most important things that helped her through this.

So there I was, trying to keep her positive. I am not a positive person, especially compared to Terri, but during this time, I tried as hard as I could. Actually, though, more than once I wondered if I was really being positive or just trying to convince both of us of what I wanted to believe. I think sometimes there's a thin line between being negative and being realistic.

We tried to keep a positive front to the kids. I sometimes think this may have had mixed results. You want them to know how bad a situation is, but they're your kids, and you want to protect them from bad things. I know now that they did understand the seriousness of the matter, but I wondered sometimes, during some of the hardest days, if I should tell them more. I think I just wanted someone to talk to about how hard it was getting to keep a positive outlook.

I tried to spend as much time as I could with Terri, as I was afraid that maybe our time together was running out. I usually got up around four A.M. and tried to get some work done. When she awoke, I tried to do whatever she needed to make her comfortable. She could never sleep late during the week, as she had radiation treatments around eight A.M. They wore her out, due to the pain, and we would come home and she would take her medicine and rest.

Some days I just sat there while she slept, thinking about how life can take some crazy twists and turns. One day you're making plans, the next you're worried that the love of your life may be gone long before anyone would have imagined. Besides, I always figured I would go first, because I know I could not make it without her. So how could this be?

When the time came for the surgery, I was amazed at Terri's strength. In spite of what a drastic change for her this was going to be, she just plowed onward. Many times, I've thought that if I had to go through what she was going through, I wouldn't make it, either from lack of resolve or lack of discipline.

She had a giant pillbox, as she took numerous pills every day, all at specific times. Even with what she was going through, she was able to keep it all straight. I have trouble remembering to take a daily vitamin sometimes. I don't know how she did it.

With all the changes they were going to make to her, our lives would never be the same, especially hers. She would go from an always-moving-and-doing-something person to someone whose every move would have to be calculated to ensure it was medically okay.

I just wanted her to be healthy. I knew that together, we could handle whatever our lives were going to be.

But the tumor was gone when Dr. Drake went to operate—a genuine, authentic miracle! People all across the country, if not the world, were praying for Terri. Someone would tell someone else to add her to their prayer list, and the number of lists just grew and grew.

Is there a medical explanation for this? Did the tumor get tired and leave? Were all the X-rays, CAT scans, and analyses wrong? Which is harder to believe: that all the medical diagnoses and doctors were wrong, every one of them, or that God performed yet another one of His miracles? I know what I believe!

Before I end this, I want to be sure I thank the wonderful doctors, nurses, staff, and every other medical professional and volunteer who always made us feel that we were getting the best care there was. These people have that extra something, and I wonder sometimes how those dealing with deadly diseases can be so upbeat and comforting all the time. God bless them!

Now that the cancer has come and gone, I have to say that going through such an ordeal is tougher on the spouse and other family members than you would think. My heart goes out to all those who suffer from this evil disease, but also to their spouses, children, siblings, parents, and other family members. It affects everyone close to the sick person, and they need prayer too.

Coming out of this, I found an inner strength in myself that I didn't know I had. I also found a sense of peace that is difficult to explain, other than to say that the peace and *grace of God comforted me. I am eternally grateful, and I am so happy that He let us keep Terri!*

—Warren Scruggs

My Man

Reaching out of distress, showing care and openness,
Wrapping around to embrace, helping to clean the mess,
Hands coming from the man I love, always by my side,
He is always there for me, taking care of his bride.

The security of his love keeps me going each day.
My love for him reaches beyond any words I can say.
His manner of seeing to my needs means everything.
I don't know how I could live without him by my side.

And the peace of God, which passeth all understanding, shall keep your hearts and minds through Christ Jesus.

—Philippians 4:7

Warren never once told me how the cancer that was in me affected the heart in him. I remember asking once. He had no response. He gave me the precious gift of strength. He gave me the courage I needed to get through the months of therapy. He let me lean on him, without fear.

Tell Me

What are you thinking about this cancer that is in me?
Does it hurt you to know that I may have to leave?
There are times when I want you to release the fear,
Yet how would I react to you being scared and in tears?

Why you gave me your strength is beyond understanding.
How could I have survived without your bearing?
Such a godly man had to be leaning on Him.
No other way could you have found this determination.

Your resolve to stay strong for me was such a blessing.
It had to be hard for you, yet you kept to the mission.
How understanding and affectionate you have been.
I am so proud and thankful to have you as my husband.

Have not I commanded thee? Be strong and of a good cour-
age; be not afraid, neither be thou dismayed: for the Lord
thy God is with thee whithersoever thou goest.
—Joshua 1:9

Because my husband is so special to me, I want to share
a poem I wrote to him.

Before I Met You

Before anyone did anything,
I met you

Life could not have existed
Before I met you

The stars were lonely
Before I met you

The clouds were gray
Before I met you

How could I have existed
Before I met you?

My thoughts cannot remember
Before I met you.

Because now I can fly, I can see, I can live
Since I met you.

*My heart is fixed, O God, my heart is fixed: I will sing and
give praise.*
—Psalm 57:7

The rest of my support came from other family members,
including my siblings, my parents, and the friends I told.

I wouldn't know what to do without my parents. They
were with me throughout the entire ordeal. When I found
out I had cancer, I worried about the two of them more than

my health. I know it was hard on them since the only other child of theirs who had cancer had died from it.

I tried to soften the blow by telling them about it on the phone. And I always tried to keep the pain inside me when I was around them, or anyone else for that matter. I loved their weekly visits and especially appreciated the rhubarb pie and the chicken and dumplings. My mother is the best cook on earth, and she knows those are my favorites.

They took good care of me and kept my mind off the cancer, which is what I needed. Without a doubt, I know I have the best parents in the world. I love them so much, and I sure know they love me.

Most of my brothers and sisters were very good to me during the fight. It really touched my heart when my little sister came by for the first time after she found out I had cancer. I was pretty drugged up and was dealing with a bit of pain that night. She started crying, and I knew my "tough act" wasn't working with her. I told her not to worry about me, that even if the cancer got me, I would be going to a better place. I also tried kidding around a bit to take the fear away from her. She saw through it all.

Some of my other siblings visited with me a bit and helped my husband out by bringing us dinners.

I think the sister who was there for me the most was Mary Ann. She came by my home all the time and called me on the phone whenever she was out of town. She made sure our food situation was always taken care of.

The week of the surgery, she gave me a couple of Christian medals that meant a lot to me. The day before the surgery, she came over and we had a nice sisterly talk. When I arrived at the hospital, she was right there, waiting with my parents. I have to say, she definitely gave me the support I needed when I required it the most.

My cousin Katrina had breast cancer a few years before I had cancer, and she gave me all of her wigs and hats to use if my hair fell out. It never did, but it helped me to know those were there for me.

My Aunt Margaret brought me her homemade strawberry pie, which is the best in existence.

I tried not to get the word of my cancer out to my friends because I didn't want them to worry. The ones who knew helped me with meals, offered their time, and gave me "surprise baskets."

Everyone was so good to me, and I appreciate it so much!

Carrying Me

They came to my aid when I needed it most.
I did not have to request their assistance.
I tried to be physically powerful around others.
I did not want anyone to worry about my cancer.

They gave me all the support I needed.
Their concern was obvious in the tears they shed.
For the first time in my life, I needed complete help.
So boldly, they came from all directions to ease my doubt.

It is of the Lord's mercies that we are not consumed, because his compassions fail not. They are new every morning: great is thy faithfulness.

—Lamentations 3:22-23

A Godly Story

Once upon a time, there was a little girl who loved her mom very much. She loved dressing in her clothes and putting on her lipstick. This little girl sometimes sat calmly across the room and watched her mom creating clothes out of nothing.

Sundays were about dressing in your best clothes, going to church, and spending time with the family while Mom oversaw everything.

This little girl's mom spent hours with a little paint-brush, putting gold leaf over scenes of the Stations of the Cross.

Whenever a member of the family had a birthday, Mom took loving care to make the day ever so special. Her daughter loved watching her magically transform a birthday cake into a masterpiece. As the cameras flashed, everyone sang "Happy Birthday," then enjoyed the special meal she had tenderly fixed.

When the school day was over, the little girl was always excited to see her mom outside waiting for her.

She enjoyed lots of picnics and barbeques too.

One day the little girl broke her leg, and her mom took good care of her, even spending the night with her at the hospital, telling her the time repeatedly all night long.

Mom was there at every piano concert, every band concert, and every parent-teacher night.

The little girl used to watch in wonder as her mom painted pictures on blank canvases.

This little girl knew she was the daughter of the best mom on earth. No other mom could possibly be so perfect. She taught her daughter how to take care of others and how to take care of herself. She taught her that God is important and prayers are essential.

As this little girl grew up, she knew her mom would always be there for her, no matter what. Her mom took pride in herself and spread this pride throughout her family.

When the girl became a woman, she tried to be the same caring mom she knew her mother to be. She was proud of her mom and loved her even more with each passing day. This woman came to realize that her mom was her hero, no doubt about it.

One day God told this woman that He would soon be taking her mom from her. She prayed that would not happen, not yet. Her inner being hurt with pure agony, and her face was soaked with tears. The woman became a little girl again, wanting to hold on to her mom forever.

And the city had no need of the sun, neither of the moon, to shine in it: for the glory of God did lighten it, and the Lamb is the light thereof.

—Revelation 21:23

Chapter 9

Dependability:
God is securing my every step

With the help of strangers, I was determined to reach the top.
I realized that God was at my side, securing my every step.
There were days when I fell and He helped me get back up.
He led me out of the strife and into His arms of love.

There was a three-month period when I needed home nursing care twice a day. I'm not sure how many different nurses came to my house, but there had to be about twenty. They were all very kind and took good care of me.

Home Nurses

I found angels on earth amid these nurses.
They have hearts that build treasures.
They are dedicated beyond expectation.
Never did I listen to a solitary objection.

You might say they were just doing their duty.
But I know they went beyond the mandatory.
Every one of them made me feel important.
I found gold care bars in each of their hearts.

They gave my wound excellent attention.
Their stories kept my mind off my condition.
Their visits were always optimistic.
Their cheerfulness kept my spirits up.

I think the conversations that were the best
Were the ones about our families and of Christ.
I enjoyed getting to know these special women.
God has their hearts in the palm of His hand.

I can do all things through Christ which strengtheneth me.
—Philippians 4:13

The radiation caused my wound to heal slowly, and I began to grow impatient. I wanted this step to be finished. Yet, no matter how long this step was going to take, I couldn't complain. It was supposed to be so much worse!

Just Fix It

The wound is giving me trouble.
It doesn't seem to want to recover.
How can I cause this wound to seal?
I am tired of waiting for it to heal.

Does someone know how to fix it?
I am tired of the length of the wait.

Vitamins, protein, and patience,
Those are the main ingredients.

I discovered that when I spoke of the incident
To the right nurse who took care of the hurt,
The two of us shared our love of God.
Within just a month, the wound healed.

*For I will restore health unto thee, and I will heal thee of
thy wounds, saith the Lord.*
—Jeremiah 30:17

Blessings can come from unexpected places. Throughout my life, I have consistently fallen in my Christian walk. I'm sure God knew I needed help. Therefore, He provided a strong hand to keep me upright.

One of my nurses, Trudi, became a dear Christian friend. Up until Thanksgiving, we had shared very little. She was one of my night nurses, and we were both very tired by the time she got there.

Sometime in early November, I began telling the other nurses about my miracle. One night, during the week of Thanksgiving, I told Trudi about it. She asked many questions, and we talked more about it every time she came over. We both loved talking about it, and about God, and about all He means to us.

During that month, we grew closer together as sisters in Christ. We never called each other or visited outside of the official visits. But I told my husband around Christmastime that I thought Trudi and I were going to become good friends.

On January 2, 2004, I had my last visit from the home nurses. Within a couple of weeks, Trudi and I were exchanging e-mails and phone calls. Over the following months, I visited her church and she visited mine. Our conversations always centered on God. I believe He brought the two of us together for a reason.

Trudi

Just a little shy, yet full of heavenly direction,
Performing her job, yet serving God with devotion,
She was determined to see that my body would heal
While she took time to exercise my spiritual will.

I told her of the miracle and His path that I was on.
In her, I found a friend with whom I can always depend.
She told me of her love and belief in Jesus Christ.
Her genuine words made me sure of my course.

It became obvious that God put the two of us together
To share His love and help each other navigate the river.
Never have I been capable of thanking Him adequately
For this seed he planted for me to share my journey.

He knew I needed someone to help me learn,
Who would listen deeply to all He was teaching me,
Showing where I was and where I needed to be.
She is my sister in Christ on every step of my new life.

A stranger not long ago, yet a sister forever more.
I will never be able to thank God enough for this gift

He gave me while I was learning to walk with Him.
God told me, "This is my gift to you, for all time!"

Verily I say unto you, If ye have faith as a grain of mustard seed, ye shall say unto this mountain, Remove hence to yonder place; and it shall remove; and nothing shall be impossible unto you.

—Matthew 17:20

How could I possibly think that this cancer would ever return? I've had several CAT scans, and none of them have shown any cancer in me. Yet the fear of its return is still there. It is easy to fall into the trap of being scared of the unknown.

Trudi has helped me get through those times. I never told anyone but her, God, and my doctors about my fear that the cancer will return. It certainly is a blessing to have her to confide in. God makes sure I always have my friend's shoulder to lean on.

Afraid

Please tell me it won't return.
I don't want to go through it again.
I cannot think clearly any longer.
My mind is full of fear.

Please bring back the trouble-free time,
When life was like a flower's bloom.

91

I want my existence always to be sunny.
I do not want the storm clouds to hurt me.

Please cleanse my body.
Make a barrier against burglary.
Tell the cancer it is not wanted.
The thought of it has me terrified.

*He giveth power to the faint; and to them that have no might
he increaseth strength.*
—Isaiah 40:29

God has prepared a path for me. I left behind all my goals and now live totally for Him. It's hard to talk to others about this. I've been accused of "getting a big head" about my relationship with my God. Some tell me I've taken it too far, that I'm not the same as I used to be. I've even been laughed at.

God knew I needed someone I could talk to who would not judge me, someone I could share my prayers with, someone who would listen to my excitement for the Lord and share her own with me.

He gave me a friend who is different from any friend I have ever known. It's hard to explain, but it's all God. We are both happily married, and our husbands are very understanding of this friendship. I'm not sure anyone else understands it, but that doesn't matter.

Trudi has given me something that no one has ever given me. She is sharing her love for God with me by helping me walk on my path with Him in a more secure way. She listens to me, prays about me, and prays with me.

She cries with me, laughs with me, and lets me lean on her. She lets God talk through her. She teaches me about God. She gives me support. She is truly my sister in Christ. I try to give her all that she gives me.

I've always known there are different kinds of love I can have for others: the love I have for my parents and siblings, the love I have for my children, the love I have for my friends, the love I have for my husband, and the love I have for God. But I didn't realize there was another type of love. You see, I love Trudi as a friend, but even more, I love her for her deep commitment to God.

It's hard to explain, but it is important for me to share what God has given me since the cancer. He gave me three very important gifts: an awesome miracle, a new life with Him, and a new sister (Trudi). Let me share my friend, my sister in Christ, with you.

There Is A Friend

This is a special friend, who causes my spirit to grow,
Whose love and praise of God causes my soul to glow.
A person whom others would think I've known for years
Just by the way she uses Scripture to calm my fears.
She is a friend beyond belief, a friend given by God.

There are days when I try to second-guess what we have.
I don't understand why I do that; it's pretty naïve.
I need to look at this friendship as what it is:
Just a sample of what waits for us beyond heaven's gates.
Nothing so pure, so simple could be anything but blessed.

There is a friend I have very close to my heart.
This friend is mine today and even after we part.
There are no words to explain how much she means to me.
If so, I would write them down right now for all to see.
I thank her for sharing this sisterhood in Christ.

For where your treasure is, there will your heart be also.
—Luke 12:34

Those who know me know that I am never at a loss for words. I believe that a friendship that has God as its foundation is worth sharing with others. That's why I feel the need to share this, as silly as it may seem to some.

Trudi, My Friend

Of all the friends I have ever met,
You are the one I will never forget.

Life without you just wouldn't be right.
I could not get through each day and night.

When life takes that crazy turn,
You are always there to help me learn.

We have shared our lives and prayers together.
I know we will be best friends forever.

When we are old and gray,
You and I will still talk every day.

You are my sister, my friend.
We will be together until the end.

If I should die before you do,
I will be in heaven, waiting for you.

The Lord that is faithful, and the Holy One of Israel, *and he shall choose thee.*
—Isaiah 49:7

The road since my miracle has been full of many tests and trials. Trudi has been right there with me through all of them. I need to highlight a few of the things God has given me recently.

The first time I visited Trudi's church, Higher Ground Baptist Church, I felt blessed by the Holy Spirit. Through that service, I met another woman who was fighting cancer. Her name is Kathy, and she is now with Christine in heaven. She was an awesome Christian and left behind a loving family and a multitude of friends. I enjoyed knowing her the last year of her life. I have great respect for her strength and courage. The few times I talked to her will always be an important part of my memories.

But the wisdom that is from above is first pure, then peaceable, gentle, and easy to be intreated, full of mercy and good fruits, without partiality, and without hypocrisy.
—James 3:17

One day, soon after this service, Trudi introduced me to her Sunday school teacher, Norma. Norma invited me to join a fantastic interdenominational, international Bible study group.

The next group meeting was on a Wednesday, but I decided that if Norma didn't call me about it, I wouldn't go. On Tuesday night, a few minutes after nine, my husband asked me if I was going to the Bible study. I told him no, because Norma hadn't called. Not even one minute later, the phone rang. It was Norma, asking if I was going. I went.

That Bible study was definitely a gift from God. It taught me the truth He wanted me to know so I could serve Him better. He showed me how important Scripture is to His teachings. On a weekly basis, this class gives me the information I need in order to serve God better. If Trudi hadn't introduced me to Norma, I would never have joined this wonderful group.

One important lesson God gave me was in the book of Habakkuk. This book has taught me to give myself totally to God and trust Him completely. Through this teaching God gave me a lesson in trust.

I have found that the power of a promise reaches inward. God is my power, and He reaches inward to give me His grace and bring out His love to others. What God told me through the book of Habakkuk is, "You need to be humble and to walk by faith. My ways are higher than your ways, so trust in Me."

Behold, his soul which is lifted up is not upright in him: but the just shall live by his faith.
—Habakkuk 2:4

Since I met Trudi, the devil has been working to destroy our friendship. We've been aware of this and have been fighting him, with God at our side.

One time the devil found a way to bring words from a mutual friend between us. It hurt badly and kept us apart, each of us thinking the other did not want to continue the friendship. We both prayed and leaned on others for help. Almost two days went by before we finally talked to each other and took care of the problem. It was a major obstacle and we had to get past it. The grace of God brought us through it.

I know the devil thought he had destroyed our friendship, but our love for God is too strong. Satan can't win something he has already lost!

Usually, when Satan tries to interfere with my life, I get very frustrated. So I looked up the definition of that word and learned that *frustrate* means "to prevent from accomplishing a purpose or fulfilling a desire; thwart." Sounds like the devil at work to me!

Consistently, God has been showing me how to defeat the devil in my life. Now I feel that the more the devil crosses my path, the better my work for God must be!

Blessed is the man that endureth temptation: for when he is tried, he shall receive the crown of life, which the Lord hath promised to them that love him.

—James 1:12

God is taking my soul in His hands and teaching me the importance of praying *with* Him. He led me to a system of prayer and fasting. I found that when I fast, my prayer becomes a cup of tender grace that touches me more deeply than anything ever has.

He even blessed my life with something I have never experienced. He gave me a prayer partner! Praying with Trudi has made my individual prayer life far more enriching.

In my Bible study, we have been discussing how we should spend extra time with God. Through prayer, our lives become closer to Him. The more time I take for God and prayer, the more at peace my mind is.

The power of the Holy Spirit provides the nurturing of our faith. Through our total belief in the truth, we are able to release ourselves to His care.

Evening, and morning, and at noon, will I pray, and cry aloud: and he shall hear my voice.
—Psalm 55:17

There came a time when my prayers were empty. There was nothing there. Everything I had been feeling the months before left me. I wasn't hearing God; I wasn't feeling Him. I started doubting Him, focusing on all the unanswered prayers.

This really hit me hard. I began thinking about all the people I had talked to that week who had treated me differently because of my excitement for God. And there were a lot of them.

A few days into this emptiness, God showed me that my fears were simply Satan messing with my exposed faith. God "left" me for a couple of days so I could work through all these questions. They needed to come out, and

I needed to work through them for the purification of my trust in Him.

The thoughts that came out of me during this time were nothing less than sin. The only way to extract them was to bring them to the surface. It embarrasses me that I let the fact that God was not talking to or touching me turn into such an act of rebellion. He told me that this was the only way I would learn. This was His way of freeing me from this sin that was still inside me, even though I didn't know it was there.

I felt like everything I had tried to do that year had turned out wrong and that I wasn't doing anyone any good. I felt like every person I had grown close to that year was just using me. I forgot all those fantastic things that had happened and let Satan take total control.

I cannot believe I let all that happen!

God told me that I needed to know what life was like without Him. I needed to rid myself of doubt and to understand what the word *trust* means as far as He is concerned.

I was upset at myself for falling from His grace. Trudi had given me some tapes to listen to earlier in the week, and I found time to listen to them on the last day of my lesson. These tapes helped me realize what I was going through. God will at times "leave" us if He sees that we need it.

Shortly after that, she happened to come by. She could see that something was troubling me, so she prayed for me. Once again, Trudi helped bring me out of Satan's hold. This was a hard lesson that God taught me. Yet it helped me to grow into a stronger Christian.

And Joshua said unto the people, Sanctify yourselves:for to morrow the Lord will do wonders among you.

—Joshua 3:5

I have spent some of my free time volunteering on the cancer floor of my local hospital, talking with cancer patients. There I met a man who was dying of lung cancer. A few weeks before, he had accepted Jesus into his life. He confided in me that he was nervous about dying. He knew he would be leaving this earth within the next few days.

I talked to him about heaven and God. He was so excited! After a few hours, I left him with his sister. I knew he wanted to live through that night.

I went back the next morning to see if he had made it, and sure enough, he had. He was sleeping while I was there, but his sister told me that he was excited about meeting his Savior. He went to heaven the following Monday.

I also met a woman about my age who was dying from cancer. We talked about Jesus and heaven. She knew that soon she would be with her father, who had died a few years earlier.

A week later, when I went to see her, she was in a coma. Before I entered the room, I asked God to use my words in any way that would help this family, and He did.

Her family was upset, but they had accepted that she would be leaving soon. I told her husband that I had heard that people who are in comas could hear what other people say to them, they're just not able to talk back. I suggested that he explain to her that the family was fine with her going on to heaven. I told him she was probably just holding on because she loved them all so much and didn't want to leave. He told me he had never thought of that and would do it.

A few days later, she left to be with Jesus. Praise God!

I have met some people through mission work whom I have invited to visit my church. It thrills my soul when I see these people at church! I've seen many people accept Jesus into their lives right in front of me, just because God put me in their path.

God has given us all a light that we need to share with others. This is all I live for. I just love God so much!

Serve the Lord with gladness: come before his presence with singing.
—Psalm 100:2

I found myself at a crossroads within a year of my miracle. I made a decision that some who are close to me didn't agree with.

I had been talking to God for months about it and finally made the decision I thought best. I didn't talk to anyone but God about this because I wanted it to be a decision only between Him and me. I even asked Him to show me a few signs to confirm I was doing the right thing, and sure enough, He handed answers to me in plain English.

When I told my husband and Trudi about this, they were excited for me. They had been holding my hand throughout the process because others whom I love dearly just didn't understand. I respect their opinions, yet I pray they will soon appreciate the truth.

I had to get away for a couple of days to spend some quality time with God. I put my life on hold for forty-eight hours and gave it all to Him. I spent those two days mainly in prayer. For a long time, He listened to all my crying and hurt. He held on to me throughout and let me talk about everything that was bothering me. I felt His touch go through my soul, reassuring me.

I fell to my knees and bowed before Him. His joy filled my being, giving me a peace I had never known. He reminded me that He will always protect me, that it is through Him that I live. He told me to keep my faith dear to my heart and His Word in front of my eyes.

Through this prayer, I left behind all my pains and felt ready to face the world I live in. If there is one thing I've learned, it is that when you give God your troubles, He takes perfect care of you. My life is in His hands, and I totally trust Him.

Then said Jesus unto his disciples, If any man will come after me, let him deny himself, and take up his cross, and follow me.
—Matthew 16:24

Since I had cancer, I have grown so deep in my faith that I cannot get enough of my dear Lord. I remember praying to Him a few years ago with a request that was deep in my heart and soul. I asked Him for a friend like no other. One who would understand me and let me share my life with her without judgments and with support. I wanted a friend I could share my love of Him with, one who would listen and share her own love for Him with me. Someone who would be a best friend and who would believe in every value I did.

He not only blessed me with an awesome miracle, but He gave me an answer to this prayer of so many years ago. He placed her in my life and told us both to enjoy!

Continue in prayer . . . with thanksgiving.
—Colossians 4:2

I was in prayer with God one day in late spring when the Holy Spirit led me to something I had never thought of, something that changed my life. It was to pray with Trudi. Now, Trudi and I had prayed together many times, but never in deep prayer.

I talked to her about it. With God's direction, we decided that we both needed to pray out loud (taking turns), to learn from each other while honestly and deeply praying to Him. So I went to her house and we nervously began doing together what we both normally did alone. This felt a bit strange at first, but as the prayers began coming out of us, we both became more comfortable. Before long we were on our knees, praising Him. Since then, we try to pray together at least once a week.

I have found that when I involve Trudi in my prayer time, I get a closer and more direct feeling of the Holy Spirit within me. We spend time reading Scripture before prayer and praise God during prayer. We ask for His direction in our lives and release our sins for His forgiveness.

I cannot count the times we have fought Satan through prayer. Our family and friends are frequently part of our prayers.

I thank God that He gave me someone on this earth I can share my love for Him so deeply with.

Prayer

We pray to and praise our Lord for He is righteous.
We thank our Father for giving His only Son, Jesus.
His forgiveness of our sins is a pure and holy truth,
Our faces are on the floor in deep reverence of His touch.

Overtaking the room - the Holy Spirit enters our prayer.
We cling to each other as we walk into His eternal care.
We talk deeply to our Lord in the spirit of our souls,
Giving Him all of our existence, for He is tremendous.

We will praise Him repeatedly, as His love endures forever.
Through prayer, we build the walls that defeat evil.
He is faithful to us; He will protect us all the while.
He said, "When two gather in My name, there am I."

*Be careful for nothing; but in every thing by prayer and
supplication with thanksgiving let your requests be made
known unto God. And the peace of God, which passeth all
understanding, shall keep your hearts and minds through
Christ Jesus.*
                                        —Philippians 4:6-7

A Godly Story

Once upon a time, there was a little girl named Hope
who loved to ride the swings. Down the street from her
house was a park, and it had the best swings in town. Every
Saturday, Hope went to this park and waited for her turn
on the swings. She rode them up and down for hours and

hours, trying to touch the sky with her feet. It was such fun! She knew she would never reach the sky, but it was a challenge trying.

As the years passed, Hope didn't go to the park as much. But every so often, she stopped by and spent a few minutes reaching for the sky.

One day she took her friend Joy with her to the park. Hope got on the swing and told Joy to join her. Both of them started swinging, trying to touch the sky with their toes. Suddenly Joy stopped and got off her swing. She told her friend to stop and get off too. Hope didn't want to, but she did anyway.

She asked her friend what was wrong. Joy smiled and told her that she knew how to truly touch the sky. Hope looked at her with excitement and asked how. Joy took her friend's hand and told her to close her eyes. Joy looked up to the sky and started praying. They began talking to God together, sharing their love for Him and bonding the depths of their friendship.

God got so much pleasure from this conversation that He blessed them with His grace. That instant they fell to their knees and bowed down in humble adoration. Their praise and love for Him energized their souls.

Soon after their prayer was over, Hope looked at her friend Joy and said, "You were right. We did touch the sky, didn't we?"

For where two or three are gathered together in my name, there am I in the midst of them.

—Matthew 18:20

Chapter 10

His World:
My life will never be the same

I began to realize that my life would never be the same,
That God had a plan for me to show others His pure love.
Since that day, I cannot get enough of my dear Lord.
Once again, He has given me life and opened my eyes.

Whether you call it transformation, evolution, change, or growth, it's all about becoming *you*, and isn't that the best kind of freedom? Could I have this feeling for the rest of my life? I've heard people say that before his downfall, a man's heart is proud. I believe I fit into that area.

I spent a lot of time setting goals and doing all I could to reach them. In the middle of all that I had planned, cancer came in and stopped every one of them in their tracks. Through the cancer, God taught me that there is much more to life than personal contentment. The real goal is to serve God the way He wants it done.

After the doctors had finished with my wound, I finally found my freedom. I saw a new world that seemed so special. God now has total control of my every move and I just love it!

New World

There was a day that I thought I had touched the sky.
There was a time when my mind had quit asking why.
I have never known such a complete sense of peace -
Never walked through the world at such a simple pace.

Through everything that almost destroyed my life,
I grew closer to my dear Lord and away from strife.
My life changed - I knew nothing would be the same.
I could not look back at my cancer, that life of pain.

My Lord gave me a new world outside the open door.
My heart smiles as my soul lies face down on the floor.
I want nothing more in life than to praise and serve Him.
He lifts my soul as I bow in deep, humble admiration.

His soul shall dwell at ease; and his seed shall inherit the earth.
—Psalm 25:13

People I love dearly have told me I've gone to the extreme. But I could never go too far for my dear Lord. I am stepping through open doors that I used to pass by, but it's all for Him. I will do anything He asks me to do. I know He would never ask me to do more than I could handle.

This year has been a learning process for me. I've made many mistakes, but I'm trying to learn from them.

The Vision

My sight is not lost; it is renewed.
I feel the vision that God has given me.

I will share His love and His goodness
With every person whose path I cross.

I need to learn lessons and to listen to signs.
I want to praise Him and give Him my service.

Sanctify the Lord God in your hearts: and be ready always to give an answer to every man that asketh you a reason of the hope that is in you with meekness and fear.
—1 Peter 3:15

Have you ever thought about how God sees us? If we could look at life through His eyes, what would we see? If you really put your mind to seeing every human being as an individual, observing every struggle and every laugh, you'd feel a deep sense of love and parental care toward them.

In God's eyes, we are His little children, and He tries to help us deal with life. We could look at the fourth commandment another way. I think it is also telling us to honor God, our heavenly Father. In His eyes, the possibilities are endless. I strive to find the place He wants me to be. I want to be a sparkle in His eyes.

How I Feel

Jesus Christ is my Lord and Savior.
His dying breath brought me here.
All of my life I will sing songs
Of His sacrifice and love for us.

Early in the morning I look up to Him,
Raising both of my arms toward heaven.
I praise my Redeemer from within my heart.
I know that His presence will never part.

I owe Him my entire life, my total soul.
I will follow Him where He tells me to go.
When I stumble on the path He has me on,
He will lift my shoulders from the ground.

Jesus is the one on whom I can always depend
To be there for me no matter what is alleged.
There are times when Christians need to learn
Struggle can be a needed resource to strength.

Recently my life has been full of terrible hurt.
I suffered it from those whom I love most.
One day I felt my heart break from the stress.
It caused me to run away with tears on my face.

It seems like honesty can make a wound
That is unbearable when experienced.
All of it comes from a misunderstanding,
Disparity that is not a companion of caring.

This makes me want to be alone in prayer.
As it is through Him, my life will recover.
I feel I need to get away from all the strife.
I want to get closer to Jesus Christ, my life.

He is the One who will never abandon me.
I have learned that during the ignominy.
Family and friends definitely will not stay,
Yet God will forever walk along the way.

*Those things, which ye have both learned, and received,
and heard, and seen in me, do: and the God of peace shall
be with you.*
—Philippians 4:9

Through my walk with cancer, I saw that my belief in God gave me the strength I needed to get past the horrible pain I was feeling. I will never let go of the renewed faith I found through the blessed miracle He gave me.

He provided me with people to help me to keep His love alive. He brought me teachings that gave me insight in areas I had never imagined. My Father gives me opportunities to serve Him repeatedly. He is teaching me how to share His love and how to fight Satan. My dear Lord is my river of life. He flows in all of us and He is the source of our every breath.

The River Of Life

I will look at the horizon and see the river.
I will follow it through the calmest waters.
I will grasp it throughout the raging rapids.
I will follow it into my heavenly Father's arms.
I will never look back and never be afraid.

There will be days when tears flow from my heart.
Never will I look for an embankment to rest upon.
My soul praises His name and my heart aches for Him.
They give me the strength to strive for His glory.
My life belongs to Him; He is the source of my every breath.

*Humble yourselves in the sight of the Lord, and he shall
lift you up.*

—James 4:10

A Godly Story

Once upon a time, there was an angel named Grace. She spent most of her time helping others conquer mountains. One day she saw a lonely boy trying to cross a mountain full of valleys. She knew he could not receive her help unless he asked God to touch his heart.

She prayed that God would give this boy an action of love.

The next day he looked to the heavens and said, "God, I trust that You will send me the strength I need to conquer this mountain I face."

Grace was so happy! She grabbed the boy's hand and led him to the foothills of the mountain. She caused the mighty obstacle to bow.

The boy was amazed that what he thought would be climbing and falling became a walk through a path of meadows. His soul possessed an everlasting joy that spread throughout the lands.

Grace looked up and smiled, for she knew he had received a very special action of love from God.

For the Lord God is a sun and shield: the Lord will give grace and glory: no good thing will he withhold from them that walk uprightly.

—Psalm 84:11

Chapter 11

My Path:
His guidance puts joy in my life

I ask Him every day to guide me on this new path I travel.
He began giving me lessons to help me serve Him better.
I can now experience the Holy Spirit dancing inside my soul,
Joining me in shouts of praises that reach into all I do.

I am the kind of person who loves to do things my way.
God had to do something dramatic to get my attention. I
suppose that taking away a cancerous tumor overnight is
dramatic!

When I think back to how I felt that day I found out He
had given me that awesome gift, I cry in humble adoration.
I will never forget that day.

It should not take such a miracle to get us to look up.
We should want to serve our God because of who He is, not
because of something He did. I reached out my hand that
day and told Him I would follow Him wherever He wanted
me to go. I ask Him every night to hold my shoulders and

to keep me on this path with Him. I love Him and cannot get enough of my Lord.

My New Path

My road had a fork that I never thought would be there.
It was full of strife and pain that would not go away.
He gave me a new, better path to travel for Him,
One that I desire to stay on until the end of time.

I will follow the pathway that lies in front of me.
My heart rides along, wishing for a fairy-tale ending.
It is not my roadway; it is the one I was given.
His love is the catalyst controlling each action.

I found a motivation just around that corner.
It gave my heart a treasure and my soul pleasure.
I can live a secure life with my Lord Almighty
Because I know the secret and I found the way.

Signs come to me; they flow through my mind.
I have to be determined to share them as I can.
I'm caught up in it as my heart is learning patience.
I want only to show His love to all those who are lost.

In the beginning God created the heaven and the earth. And the earth was without form, and void; and darkness was upon the face of the deep. And the Spirit of God moved upon the face of the waters. And God said, Let there be light: and there was light.

—Genesis 1:1-3

Throughout my life, I have fallen on my Christian path. After this miracle, I decided that I never wanted to fall again. Well, I have a few times, but God has always been there to pick me up.

One of the most important things I've learned this year is that all of us can grow closer to God through prayer. I've spent hours in intense prayer, just to get close to Him. He is so awesome!

I've also been in several Bible studies since the cancer. His Word nurtures our knowledge of Him. I need His strength to get through each day. Satan is an evil part of all of our lives, and only through prayer can we build up our armor against him. I depend on my Lord to guide my every step.

Guided Strength

Give me the strength to do Your will, Lord.
I need You to guide me; give me knowledge.
The future holds a space with my Lord in it.
Every day, every minute, my heart is dedicated.

To share is the secret and to grow is the plan.
There's always room for more in God's loving hand.
I know that miracles are support from above.
His heart reaches in the direction of our soul.

Hold my hand, dear, sweet God; lead me on this new path.
I give You my life to nurture others and bring souls home.
I cannot do it alone; I require You and all of Your help.
I want to see the difference between reality and hope.

Thy word is a lamp unto my feet, and a light unto my path.

—Psalm 119:105

God has opened many doors for me. He has put me in awesome Bible studies to learn more about Him. He placed me in various mission areas to serve Him. He has brought people to me so I could share His love. I've shared Him with people who were dying and with some who were lost. Since I gave my life to Him, He has consistently put people in my path to share His love with. I love serving my Father in heaven!

Steps

I talked to the Lord until my eyes closed.
My mind remembered His every word.
When I awoke, my soul bowed in praise
While my eyes saw through the haze.

His words became the light of my day.
Soon I walked calmly up His pathway.
Deep in my soul, I encountered His touch.
I never knew that He loved me so much.

As the days went by, I learned more of Him.
I began to get a glimpse of His heaven.
Within months, the Bible became my attendant.
My prayers became my every manifestation.

My Path: His guidance puts joy in my life

One day I was weak and needed His hand.
Through deep prayer, I found my closest friend.
My Lord reached out to me, putting His arms
Around my soul, and He held me like a newborn.

I spent that spring stepping into knowledge.
I prepared for a summer of complete servitude.
I willingly gave Him every breath and step
As I observed souls seeking out His help.

The more time I spend as His servant,
I see that nothing else is important.
I want to be just like my dear Jesus,
My Lord, my Savior, my existence.

Recently my heavenly Father opened a door.
That first step shocked my life to its core.
I felt every emotion and cried endless tears.
Some have shunned me and tried my fears.

With Him at my side I will not stumble.
My faith is true and my soul is humble.
My eyes are closed and my hand is in His.
His light will forever guide my steps.

*Seest thou how faith wrought with his works, and by works
was faith made perfect? And the scripture was fulfilled which
saith, Abraham believed God, and it was imputed unto him
for righteousness: and he was called the Friend of God. Ye
see then how that by works a man is justified, and not by
faith only.*

—James 2:22-24

There was a day, during my cancer fight, when I was all by myself, dealing with a bundle of pain and a broken spirit. Full of medicine, I looked up to my heavenly Father and told Him I loved Him. Then I fell asleep.

That day I knew my life would never be the same. I could die. I probably would die. Yet I loved God more than life. He was in control.

Today, I still look to the heavens and tell God I love Him. Only now, I can see how my life has changed. I never knew it could be this way. Now, when I tell God I love Him, I also thank Him for the miracle of August 8 and for giving me this new life with Him.

What He Has Given Me

Once the dust had cleared,
All the wounds had healed.
I looked about and saw the meadow
That God had placed on my shadow.

My heavenly Father gave me a new life
That caused me to forget the strife.
He filled my soul with the Holy Spirit.
He gave me a special piece of His heart.

I cannot get enough of my Savior, Jesus Christ.
I yearn to show His love to countless lives.
It makes no difference what my future may hold.
All the days of my life, I will praise my dear Lord.

Then shall thy light break forth as the morning, and thine health shall spring forth speedily: and thy righteousness shall go before thee; the glory of the Lord shall be thy reward.

—Isaiah 58:8

A Godly Story

I crossed a road one day and found many curves. These curves became challenges that tested my soul. At first, they were easy to defeat, but soon they began to tug at my heart. I looked around, noticed the beauty along the path, and started spending time getting to know it. My soul leaped with gladness as I took in this beauty. The curves were still ahead, but they seemed easier to deal with once I let the beauty become part of my life.

As I discovered new and more intense beauty, the curves became more plentiful. Yet they did not seem as wide as they used to be. Every time I navigated past a curve, the beauty on the other side was more plentiful.

If the curve became too difficult, I took a few steps back into the beauty, and that helped me defeat the curve. Soon I became an experienced navigator of this road. I found the beauty in His promise, in the greatness of His love, and in the depth of His grace.

Then spake Jesus again unto them, saying, I am the light of the world: he that followeth me shall not walk in darkness, but shall have the light of life.

—John 8:12

121

Chapter 12

Responsibilities Of Reality:
Knowing and loving God

I have no doubt that there are seeds for me to spread.
Yet He requests that I water the other side of the world.
I need to open my eyes to the inner truth that touched me.
My Father commands me to be loyal; my soul leaps for joy.

Facing the depths of reality is not just a dream; it is a responsibility. He put us here for a purpose. We must live in a way that will make the world stand up and listen. If we face the realms with Him in our hearts, many lives will live forever. These saved souls must then face their destinies. Without question, the world would change, and heaven would be fuller because of it.

Being a true Christian has certainty attached to it. The future of millions of lives rests in how we choose to participate in our faith.

There was a lesson for me in all the strife I had to go through while I had cancer. God woke me up and gave me a chance to serve Him in a way I never had before. Because of how dramatic this miracle was, I finally paid attention.

I could never turn back now, because I know how fantastic it is to live my life for Him. I want everyone to feel what I'm feeling. It is a tremendous touch of grace. There are times when my soul is so overwhelmed I spend hours crying in humbleness to Him.

I Was Paying Attention

One season I crossed the valley of life,
Yet I could not get past the strife.
I felt the stars falling from the sky.
I wondered if I could touch the lie.

I saw people running to the carrot;
Even then, not filling the bucket.
The truth became less important.
The shackles began to bend to want.

Need was not part of the method.
Desire began to take command.
Nothing mattered in this false wrath.
Everyone walked the wrong path.

I looked up to the sky; I asked for relief.
The only way I knew to release this grief
Was through the Lord my God in heaven,
Who knows the best for all brethren.

As I walked down the path of truth,
I looked in the eyes of the sheltered sheep.

I saw hurt, pain, discourse, and humiliation.
I realized that I was paying attention.

I dropped to my knees and sent my request
For all these souls who haven't seen the light.
I asked for His forgiveness and blessing.
He understood and changed the journey.

For as the body without the spirit is dead, so faith without works is dead also.

—James 2:26

Seven months after the miracle, God told me through prayer that I would be going on an overseas mission trip. He told me nothing else about it. Since I've learned to have complete trust in Him, I began telling others about this mission trip. When they asked me, "Where?" I replied, "God hasn't told me yet."

A few weeks later, the Holy Spirit led me to join a local missions group that was supposed to lead me to my overseas trip. I checked out all the local missions I could find and never felt like any were where He wanted me to be. Finally, I checked to see if my own church had one; sure enough, it did, and I felt God tell me that it was the one. I joined and began training to help families around town deal with food and money problems.

In my second week of training, I met with the leader of the group. She asked me why I had decided to join. I told her that God wanted me to go on an overseas mission trip and then led me to join their group to prepare for it. She looked at me as if I had lost my mind.

She pulled out a piece of paper and told me, "I have an opportunity to go on one of two mission trips: either to Hungary or a domestic one. I was the final person chosen for the Hungary trip. One of the group leaders needed my decision today. Well, this morning I chose the domestic trip." She looked at me, handed me the sheet of paper, and said, "I think this one is for you."

I looked at the piece of paper; it had the information for the Hungary trip on it.

She then took me to the church that was sponsoring this trip. It just happened to be the church where I'd been attending Sunday night services. They accepted me into the group, saying it was definitely "a God thing." I made a small deposit on the cost of the trip.

Imagine the faces of my family and friends when I told them how God told me where I would be going on my mission trip!

The trip was in October, so I spent the time in between preparing. God was constantly giving me lessons, including how to pray. I dedicated the months before the trip to my heavenly Father and did the best I could to honor Him.

A few weeks before the trip, I needed to turn in the final $800 of the cost of the trip. I didn't have the money and figured I would have to tell those in charge that I couldn't go. It was hard for me to admit that I was going to let God down this way. So I prayed about it.

A few days before the money was due, a member of the sponsoring church came to me and handed me the full amount in cash! I gave it back and said it was too much money for me to take. This person told me that God said to give it to me for the mission trip, that I needed it because He wanted me to go. I couldn't say no to that! I accepted the money with a humble heart. Praise God that He covers every angle when He is using a person for His glory.

For God, who commanded the light to shine out of darkness, hath shined in our hearts, to give the light of the knowledge of the glory of God in the face of Jesus Christ.
—2 Corinthians 4:6

Eight other people were taking this mission trip. We were going to have a conference for Hungarian women. Each of the female members of our mission team was responsible for teaching at least one class. My class was about cancer and prayer.

I prayed alone to God for more than four hours the afternoon of my class. I asked Him to use my tongue any way He wished, to help me speak well enough so the translator could understand me, to allow many women to come to my class, and for at least one Hungarian woman to accept Jesus into her heart that night.

My help cometh from the Lord, which made heaven and earth.
—Psalm 121:2

The class had a great turnout of women who either had cancer or had a family member with cancer. I witnessed to them about how God saw me through my cancer. I told them how important prayer was during this time. I explained to them that it is impossible to pray if you don't

127

know God. I told them that if any of them needed to know God, they could see me after class and I would introduce them to Him.

Come now, and let us reason together, saith the Lord: though your sins be as scarlet, they shall be as white as snow; though they be red like crimson, they shall be as wool.
—Isaiah 1:18

After I explained my trial with cancer, I asked if anyone wanted to come forward and have the class pray for her needs. Women started coming forward with prayer requests. I knelt with each one in front of the class and held her hand, with my other arm around her shoulder. Seven women came up for this prayer time, and the class prayed for whatever each need was.

Therefore with lovingkindness have I drawn thee.
—Jeremiah 31:3

After this prayer period was over, I asked for anyone who desired to have individual prayer to come to the front with the interpreter and me, and that we would pray with her. I also asked that anyone who needed to know God come forward too. I prayed with several women. When the last woman sat down, she looked at me and said, "I want to pray, but I don't know God."

I sought the Lord, and he heard me, and delivered me from all my fears.
—Psalm 34:4

I introduced her to God and talked to her about Jesus, and she accepted Him into her heart. I then prayed with her and asked our team leader to pray the sinner's prayer with her. After she gave her life to Jesus, I talked to her about going to church and studying the Word. Then we talked about prayer and how the Holy Spirit would indwell her soul.

Verily, verily, I say unto you, He that believeth on me hath everlasting life.
—John 6:47

As we were talking about the Holy Spirit, the interpreter started laughing. We looked at her with puzzled expressions. She told us we were talking to each other *without needing her to interpret!* We didn't realize it while it was happening, but God blessed this Hungarian woman and me by enabling us to understand each other's language for a few minutes!

For thou, Lord, wilt bless the righteous; with favour wilt thou compass him as with a shield.
—Psalm 5:12

This woman came to our meeting lost and left a child of God. I was so happy for her! She had only attended this class because she had cancer. I know that she is why God wanted me to go on this overseas mission trip. Praise God!

That night and the next afternoon, I spent hours in prayer. I praised God for using me in this way. I praised Him for giving this Hungarian woman life.

Thou, even thou, art Lord alone; thou hast made heaven, the heaven of heavens, with all their host, the earth, and all things that are therein, the seas, and all that is therein, and thou preservest them all; and the host of heaven worshippeth thee.

—Nehemiah 9:6

Anyone can belong to God, from today on, if he believes in Him with all his heart.

For whosoever shall call upon the name of the Lord shall be saved.

—Romans 10:13

You cross the bridge into God's family when you turn to God by asking Christ to be part of your life. There is no such thing as a one-way relationship. God did His part when His Son died for you; now it is your move.

Who his own self bare our sins in his own body on the tree, that we, being dead to sins, should live unto righteousness: by whose stripes ye were healed.

—1 Peter 2:24

Turning to God means you are also turning *from* something. When you turn to Him, you "repent." You cannot give yourself to Jesus while hanging on to the sin He died for. You need to turn your back on "my way" choices such as lying, sexual immorality, anger, etc. and begin doing things God's way.

To choose this relationship, you must do four things:

1. ADMIT your spiritual need. Confess that you are a sinner.
2. REPENT. Be willing to turn from your sin.
3. BELIEVE that Jesus Christ died for you on the cross.
4. RECEIVE Jesus Christ into your heart and life by choosing this relationship over your current life of sin and separation from Him.

Behold, I stand at the door, and knock: if any man hear my voice, and open the door, I will come in to him, and will sup with him, and he with me.
—Revelation 3:20

The Hungarian women prayed the "sinner's prayer." If you want to accept Jesus into your life, pray this prayer, or one similar to it:

My dear Lord and Savior, Jesus Christ, I know I am a sinner and I need Your forgiveness. I want to quit living my life for me and start living it for You. I believe that You died on the cross and rose from the grave in order to pay the penalty for my sins.

Oh, dear Jesus, I am sorry that my life has not been pleasing to You. I want to turn from my sins and begin a relationship with You. I invite You to come into my heart and life as my Savior and my Lord. I trust in You alone for my salvation, and I accept Your gift of eternal life.

Humble yourselves in the sight of the Lord, and he shall lift you up.
—James 4:10

131

A Godly Story

I looked up and saw a light shining in my face. I crossed the field that lay in front of me without losing sight of this immaculate light. It drew me closer until I could feel its warmth. No longer was I able to see where I had crossed.

I felt the depth of the light engulfing my heart. The light began shining through my eyes toward the sea of darkness. I fell to my knees and let the Holy Spirit take control. Life was no longer the same.

> *The spirit of man is the candle of the Lord, searching all the inward parts of the belly.*
> —Proverbs 20:27

God is the Author of the most important Book of all time: the Bible, His "owner's manual" for a human life. In His Book, He says:

> *For God so loved the world, that he gave his only begotten Son, that whosoever believeth in him should not perish, but have everlasting life.*
> —John 3:16

> *The Spirit itself beareth witness with our spirit, that we are the children of God.*
> —Romans 8:16

> *If thou shalt confess with thy mouth the Lord Jesus, and shalt believe in thine heart that God hath raised him from the dead, thou shalt be saved. For with the heart man believeth*

unto righteousness; and with the mouth confession is made unto salvation. For the scripture saith, Whosoever believeth on him shall not be ashamed.

—Romans 10:9-11

For what is a man profited, if he shall gain the whole world, and lose his own soul? or what shall a man give in exchange for his soul?

—Matthew 16:26

Gift From God

One day, when I was busy building my goals,
I looked to my side and saw them crashing down.
I looked up and said, "God, please don't let this be true."
Yet when I looked around, I learned my life had changed.

I dropped my life to fight this battle of terror.
No smiles to ease my pain, no road for the escape.
I cried for hours, not knowing what the future held.
I prayed for another chance to turn my life around.

The fight was hard and brought me down to earth.
I shed my dignity and lost my pride in the struggle.
Then I looked up past the rubble and saw the tunnel's end.
Yet I had not won the battle; my life would never be the same.

I took a deep breath and tears soaked my face.
My body did not want to accept what the future held.
My soul insisted on faith, to believe the truth.
I believed, but had never believed enough to let go.

My last day of what was left of normal came upon me.
I sat down by myself and gave my entire future away.
I looked up to the Lord my God and asked for a miracle.
I gave my life to Him and accepted His will.

I slept that night better than I had all year.
The fight had been long and I tried to calm my fear.
The next morning I took the road to the life of change.
I let my doctor take my body in her hands to repair.

What I had not known was that God repaired me first.
Yes! That day was the beginning of all I know.
The months to come were a different kind of battle.
I had to climb out of the woods and into the sunshine.

I look around and see the support He has given me:
Caring, loving people who share my love for Him.
Yet never have I been able to thank Him enough
For this miracle that gave me a new life with Him.

With the help of strangers, I was determined to reach the top.
I realized that God was at my side, securing my every step.
There were days when I fell and He helped me get back up.
He led me out of the strife and into His arms of love.

I began to realize that my life would never be the same,
That God had a plan for me to show others His pure love.
Since that day, I cannot get enough of my dear Lord.
Once again, He has given me life and opened my eyes.

I ask Him every day to guide me on this new path I travel.
He began giving me lessons to help me serve Him better.
I can now experience the Holy Spirit dancing inside my soul,
Joining me in shouts of praises that reach into all I do.

I have no doubt that there are seeds for me to spread.
Yet He requests that I water the other side of the world.
I need to open my eyes to the inner truth that touched me.
My Father commands me to be loyal; my soul leaps for joy.

To order additional copies of

CANCER
WITH
GOD

Have your credit card ready and call:

1-877-421-READ (7323)

or please visit our web site at
www.pleasantword.com

Also available at:
www.amazon.com
and
www.barnesandnoble.com

Printed in the United States
52776LVS00002B/49